Trauma and Orthopaedics at a Glance

Henry Willmott
Consultant Trauma and Orthopaedic Surgeon
East Sussex Healthcare NHS Trust
United Kingdom

WILEY Blackwell

This edition first published 2016 © 2016 by John Wiley & Sons, Ltd.

Registered Office
John Wiley & Sons, Ltd, The Atrium, Southern Gate, Chichester, West Sussex, PO19 8SQ, UK

Editorial Offices
9600 Garsington Road, Oxford, OX4 2DQ, UK
The Atrium, Southern Gate, Chichester, West Sussex, PO19 8SQ, UK
350 Main Street, Malden, MA 02148-5020, USA

For details of our global editorial offices, for customer services and for information about how to apply for permission to reuse the copyright material in this book please see our website at www.wiley.com/wiley-blackwell

Library of Congress Cataloging-in-Publication Data

Willmott, Henry, author.
  Trauma and orthopaedics at a glance / Henry Willmott.
    p. ; cm. – (At a glance series)
  Includes bibliographical references and index.
  ISBN 978-1-118-80253-3 (pbk.)
I. Title.   II. Series: At a glance series (Oxford, England)
  [DNLM: 1. Musculoskeletal Diseases–therapy.   2. Orthopedic Procedures.
3. Musculoskeletal System–injuries.   4. Wounds and Injuries–therapy. WE 140]
  RC925
  616.7–dc23
                              2014033409

A catalogue record for this book is available from the British Library.

Wiley also publishes its books in a variety of electronic formats. Some content that appears in print may not be available in electronic books.

Cover image: iStock/ © Philartphace

Set in 9.5/11.5pt Minion by SPi Publisher Services, Pondicherry, India

1   2016

Trauma and Orthopaedics
at a Glance

For Erika

This title is also available as an e-book.
For more details, please see
www.wiley.com/buy/9781118802533
or scan this QR code:

Contents

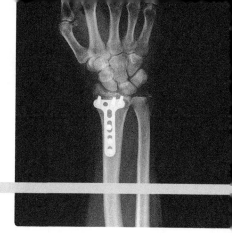

Preface

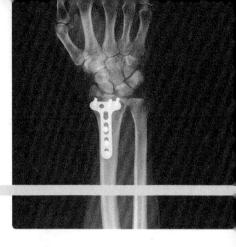

This compact book provides a general overview of the most common orthopaedic problems encountered on wards and in clinics. It is not an exhaustive tome, but will furnish the reader with key facts on which to base further reading. It is also suitable as a revision guide for medical school finals.

Orthopaedics is a fascinating and hugely varied speciality. The patients range from newborn infants to the elderly. The pathologies vary from minor aches and pains to life-threatening trauma. Orthopaedic operations are hands-on procedures, combining knowledge of anatomy and biomechanics. Working as a junior doctor in orthopaedics should be one of the best jobs of the foundation years: there is something for everyone. Those leaning towards a future in general medicine will enjoy managing the many medical conditions encountered on the ward, while those looking to a career as a GP will have the opportunity to learn about the myriad musculoskeletal injuries that we treat. Finally, those intending to pursue a career as a surgeon will have the opportunity to acquire surgical skills in theatre.

Sadly, many medical schools still spend far too little time teaching orthopaedics. This speciality is quite different from any other. The nature of the work is unique and the terminology is different. It is often the first time many foundation doctors are given significant responsibility on the wards.

In addition, new doctors will be expected to present cases in the morning trauma meetings, invariably a harrowing experience at first. Therefore many junior doctors start their foundation job feeling underprepared. This book addresses that deficit. It is aimed at senior medical students and foundation doctors, though those in other professions such as nurses, physiotherapists and occupational therapists will find it helpful. I would suggest that foundation doctors spend around 15 minutes on each chapter, and read two every day. By the end of the first month you will have read the whole book and have a good understanding of the main conditions you are likely to encounter.

I have followed the proven *at a Glance* format: full-page illustrations are paired with concise text. There are six sections: basic sciences; adult orthopaedics; paediatric orthopaedics; trauma; a section for a junior doctor in orthopaedics and finally a simple guide on performing a selected range of practical procedures. The last two sections are unique and will be helpful to those starting out in clinical orthopaedics. I have tried to use as many X-rays as possible throughout, all taken from real patients with genuine problems. The online material consists of multiple-choice questions and case studies, which will help reinforce knowledge.

I hope that this book fuels your interest in orthopaedics and helps you deliver compassionate care to your patients. Good luck and enjoy the job!

Henry Willmott

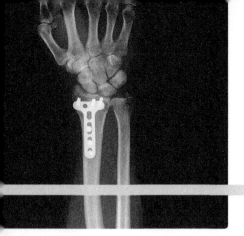

Acknowledgements

Many of the X-rays in the illustrations have been provided by colleagues. Particular thanks are due to Om Lahoti who supplied images for the paediatric section. I am indebted to Matt Stephenson who kindly put me in touch with the publishers. The editorial and production staff at Wiley have been tireless in converting my vision into reality. I am also very grateful to the illustrators who converted my cartoon-like scrawlings into professional images. Finally, I want to express my gratitude to Chris Ferguson whose critical eye and attention to detail kept my grammar and syntax on the straight and narrow!

Material is used from the following source, with permission:

Faiz O, Blackburn S & Moffat D. *Anatomy at a Glance*, 3rd edn, 2011. Wiley-Blackwell: Oxford.

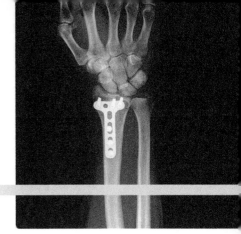

How to use your revision guide

Features contained within your revision guide

Each topic is presented in a double-page spread with clear, easy-to-follow diagrams supported by succinct explanatory text.

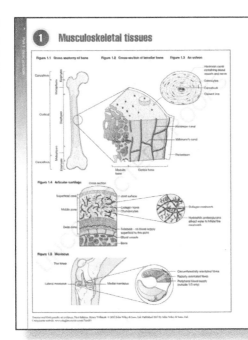

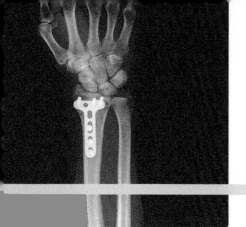

About the companion website

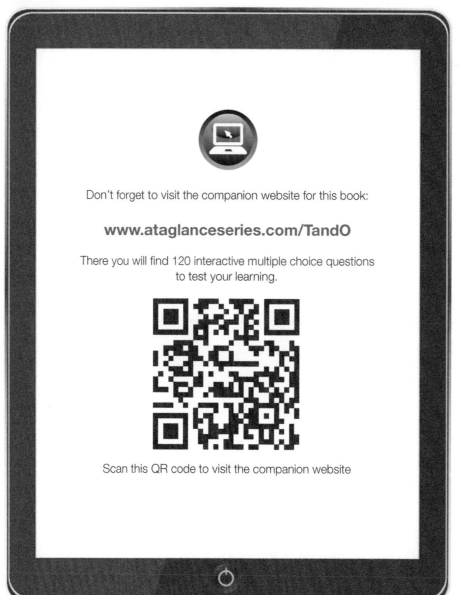

Don't forget to visit the companion website for this book:

www.ataglanceseries.com/TandO

There you will find 120 interactive multiple choice questions to test your learning.

Scan this QR code to visit the companion website

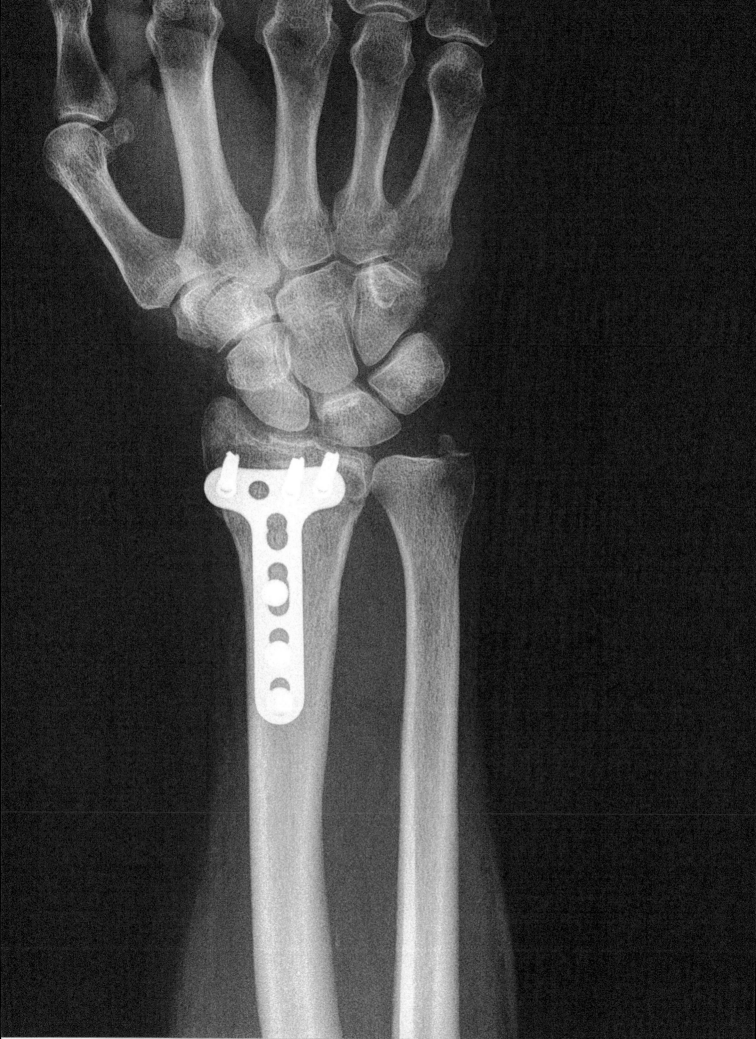

Basic sciences

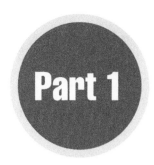

Chapters

 Visit the companion website at www.ataglanceseries.com/TandO to test yourself on these topics.

1 Musculoskeletal tissues

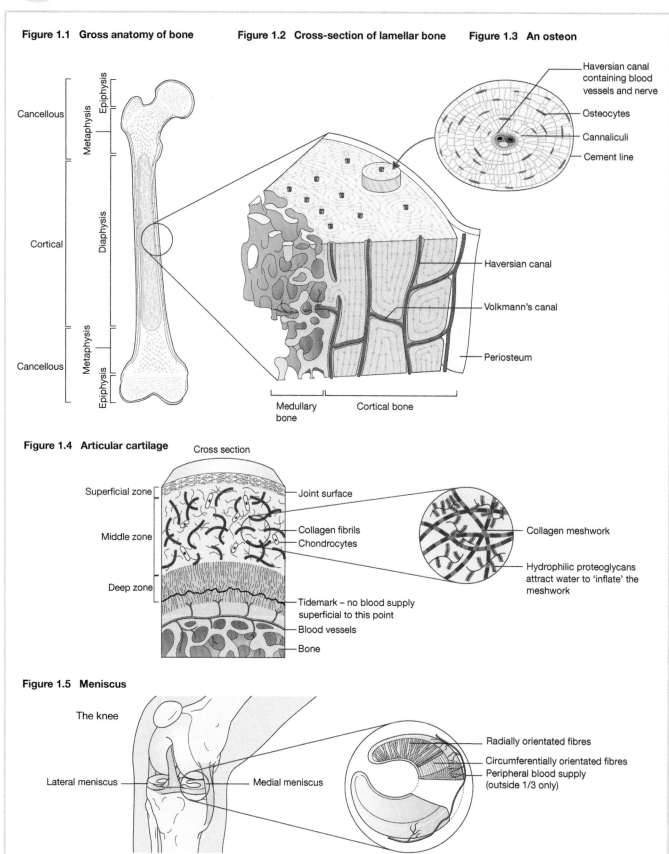

Figure 1.1 Gross anatomy of bone

Cancellous — Epiphysis / Metaphysis
Cortical — Diaphysis
Cancellous — Metaphysis / Epiphysis

Figure 1.2 Cross-section of lamellar bone

- Haversian canal
- Volkmann's canal
- Periosteum
- Medullary bone
- Cortical bone

Figure 1.3 An osteon

- Haversian canal containing blood vessels and nerve
- Osteocytes
- Cannaliculi
- Cement line

Figure 1.4 Articular cartilage

Cross section

- Superficial zone
- Middle zone
- Deep zone

- Joint surface
- Collagen fibrils
- Chondrocytes
- Tidemark – no blood supply superficial to this point
- Blood vessels
- Bone

- Collagen meshwork
- Hydrophilic proteoglycans attract water to 'inflate' the meshwork

Figure 1.5 Meniscus

The knee

- Lateral meniscus
- Medial meniscus

- Radially orientated fibres
- Circumferentially orientated fibres
- Peripheral blood supply (outside 1/3 only)

Trauma and Orthopaedics at a Glance, First Edition. Henry Willmott.
© 2016 John Wiley & Sons, Ltd. Published 2016 by John Wiley & Sons, Ltd. Companion website: www.ataglanceseries.com/TandO

Bone

Bone is living tissue and serves three functions:
- **Biochemical** – calcium and phosphate reservoir.
- **Haematological** – haemopoiesis
- **Biomechanical** – support of the limbs.
  Bone is composed of **10% cells, 90% matrix**.
- The **matrix** provides strength. It is itself composed of:
  - 40% **organic matrix** – sheets of collagen that resist tension;
  - 60% **inorganic matrix** – crystals of a compound called hydroxyapatite, which is a molecule compound of calcium and phosphate. It is good at resisting compression.
- The **cells** produce and maintain the bone and there are three types:
  - **Osteoblasts** – bone-forming cells, producing collagen.
  - **Osteocytes** – as osteoblasts lay down collagen, some become trapped within the matrix. These cells go into a dormant state, only reactivating if needed in the future.
  - **Osteoclasts** – bone-resorbing cells, derived from macrophages; they produce acid to dissolve bone. They are important for normal bone turnover and remodelling after fractures.

  There are two types of bone in the body:
- **Immature** or **woven bone**, which is found in children's growing bones and fracture callus. The arrangement of collagen fibres is random and strength is therefore low.
- **Mature** or **lamellar bone**, which is normal adult bone. The collagen fibres are highly organised into sheets (called lamellae) and therefore the bone is very strong.

Lamellar bone can be subdivided into cortical or cancellous bone:
- **Cortical bone** is the densest and strongest form and makes up the hard outer surfaces of a long bone. The lamellae are arranged in rings called osteons (see Figure 1.3).
- **Cancellous bone** is found in the centre and metaphyseal regions of long bones. It is less strong and less dense, with a 'spongy' appearance. It contains many cells.

The surface of bones is covered with **periosteum**. This is composed of an inner **cambial layer**, which is very vascular and contains many osteoblasts, contributing to circumferential growth. The outer **fibrous layer** is strong and tough. It is continuous with joint capsules and ligament insertions. In children the periosteum is very thick, which is of clinical relevance when treating fractures.

Cartilage

Cartilage is a connective tissue produced by chondroblasts. There are three main types of cartilage: fibrocartilage; elastic cartilage and hyaline cartilage. Of particular interest to the orthopaedic surgeon is **hyaline cartilage**, which lines the ends of the bones within a synovial joint.

Hyaline cartilage is composed of ground substance and cells.
- **Ground substance** is made up of:
  - **Proteoglycans**, which are large molecules consisting of multiple sugar molecules attached to a protein backbone. They are very hydrophilic and attract water to keep the cartilage turgid.
  - **Collagen** in an interlinked meshwork of long molecules. This resists shear force and the meshwork is 'inflated' by the water-attracting proteoglycans to resist compression.
- **Cells** are mainly chondrocytes, which produce the proteoglycans and collagen.

Articular cartilage is highly structured and can be divided into distinct zones (see Figure 1.4). This specialised structure resists shear at the surface, and compression at the base. As a compound structure, the cartilage functions to:
- reduce friction between joint surfaces;
- assist in producing lubricating fluid;
- distribute load evenly across the joint surface.

Cartilage is avascular, aneural and alymphatic. This means that it cannot heal itself in the event of injury. If the injury is superficial to the tidemark, no healing will occur. If the injury extends below the tidemark, bleeding will occur. The defect will go on to heal with scar tissue, which is unspecialised and poorly structured fibrocartilage. Although not as good as hyaline cartilage, it is better than having a large defect. This is the principle by which microfracture works (see Chapter 3).

Meniscus

The menisci are found within the knee joint (although similar structures are also seen in the sternoclavicular and temporomandibular joints, these are of little clinical relevance to the orthopaedic surgeon). There are two crescenteric menisci in each knee – a medial and lateral meniscus.

They are composed of fibres of fibrocartilage, arranged in longitudinal and radial bands. They serve to:
- evenly distribute load across the knee joint, especially in flexion;
- absorb impact;
- aid in stabilising the knee.

Menisci can become torn, resulting in locking and clicking of the knee joint. The menisci have a poor blood supply. In adults, only the peripheral third is vascular. Therefore, unless a tear is within this zone, it will not heal. Most meniscal tears are therefore treated by excision of the torn segment. Once part of the meniscus has been lost, greater forces are transmitted to the articular cartilage, increasing the risk of developing arthritis in the future.

Ligaments and tendons

Ligaments connect bone to bone and stabilise joints. Tendons connect muscles to bone and act to convert muscle contraction into movement.

Ligaments and tendons are composed of longitudinally aligned collagen fibres and are very strong in tension. Ligaments are slightly more elastic than tendons. Over-stretching a ligament results in a sprain.

2 Bone metabolism

Figure 2.1 Calcium and phosphate homeostasis

Figure 2.2 Manifestations of osteoporosis

Figure 2.3 Rickets

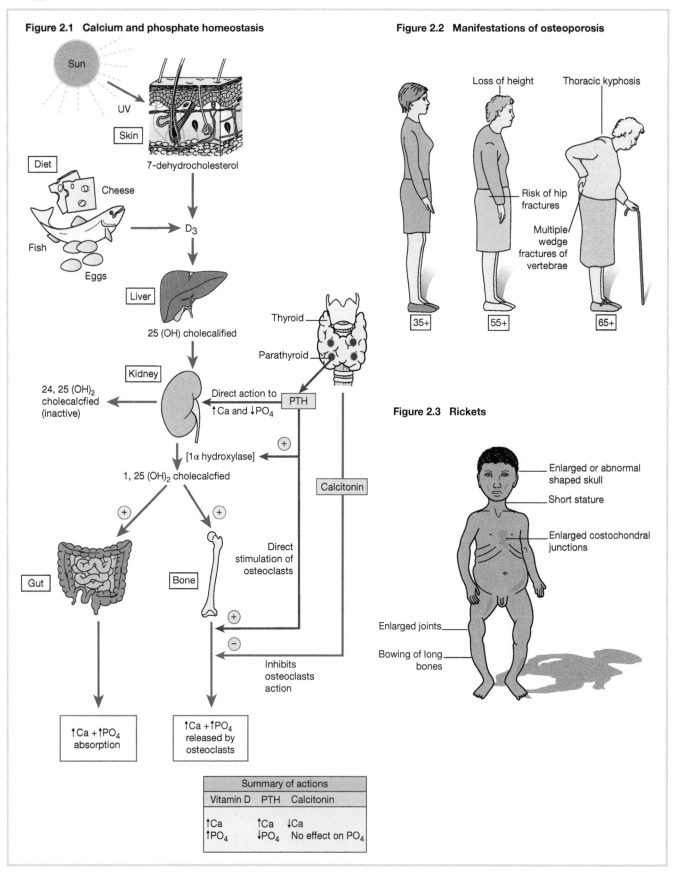

Trauma and Orthopaedics at a Glance, First Edition. Henry Willmott.
© 2016 John Wiley & Sons, Ltd. Published 2016 by John Wiley & Sons, Ltd. Companion website: www.ataglanceseries.com/TandO

Calcium, phosphate and bone mass

Calcium (Ca) is vital for muscle and nerve function. Ninety-nine percent of the body's calcium is stored within bone. Only 1% is free to circulate and half of this is bound to plasma proteins. Phosphate (PO_4) acts as a buffer for enzyme function. Eighty-five percent of phosphate is stored in bone.

Calcium and PO_4 are stored bound together in the form of hydroxyapatite: $Ca_{10}(PO_4)_6(OH)_2$. The bone cells are responsible for maintaining calcium and phosphate homeostasis. Under the control of hormones, osteoclasts break down hydroxyapatite to liberate Ca and PO_4, whereas osteoblasts lay down new hydroxyapatite, increasing bone mass and removing Ca and PO_4 from the circulation.

Bone mass is determined by the balance between osteoclastic bone resorption and osteoblastic bone deposition.

Recommended calcium intake

Calcium is found in dairy products. The required amount varies:
- Children: 600 mg/day
- Adolescents: 1200 mg/day
- Adult men and women: 750 mg/day
- Lactating women: 2000 mg/day
- Postmenopausal women: 1500 mg/day

The role of vitamin D

Vitamin D is a steroid hormone that has to be activated in order to have effect. It is found in fish oil or can be created by the action of UV light on 7-dehydrocholesterol in the skin. The resulting cholecalciferol is then hydroxylated in the liver to form 25-hydroxycholecalciferol, and is hydroxylated a second time in the kidney to form 1,25-dihydroxycholecalciferol. This is the active form. It acts on the duodenum to stimulate dietary absorption of Ca and PO_4, and also stimulates osteoclasts to breakdown hydroxyapatite. The net effect is to increase serum Ca.

The role of parathyroid hormone

Produced in the chief cells of the parathyroid glands, this hormone is released in response to low serum Ca levels. It acts directly on osteoclasts to stimulate breakdown of hydroxyapatite and the resulting release of Ca and PO_4. It also has two effects on the kidneys: it increases hydroxylation of 25-hydroxycholecalciferol to the active form; and it increases the excretion of PO_4. The net effect is to increase serum Ca and decrease serum PO_4.

The role of calcitonin

This is a hormone produced by clear cells in the thyroid in response to high serum calcium levels. It directly inhibits osteoclasts, thereby reducing serum Ca.

Other regulators

- Oestrogen prevents osteoclasts breaking down hydroxyapatite and therefore maintains bone mass.
- Corticosteroids inhibit calcium absorption from the gut and limit osteoblast activity resulting in reduced bone mass.
- Thyroxine stimulates osteoclasts and reduces bone mass.
- Smoking reduces bone mass by inhibiting osteoblasts.

Disordered bone metabolism

Osteoporosis

This is a decrease in bone mass. The structure of bone itself is normal, but there is less of it – i.e. a quantitative, not a qualitative defect (compare this to rickets, see below). Calcium and PO_4 levels are normal. The risk of fracture is increased.

Risk factors for osteoporosis include:
- Increasing age.
- Female sex.
- Late menarche, early menopause – reduced oestrogen exposure.
- Dietary deficiency of Ca or vitamin D.
- Low body mass – peak bone mass is achieved in early 20s. Anorexia at this time predicts future osteoporosis.
- Smoking and alcohol – inhibit osteoblasts.
- Family history – ask about maternal hip fracture.
- Northern European Caucasian population.

The 'strength' of bone is measured by Bone Mineral Density. It is determined by a technique known as DEXA (dual energy X-ray absorptiometry) scanning. This produces a T score and a Z score, which denote the number of standard deviations the patient's bone mass lies from either peak bone mass (T-score), or age-specific bone mass (Z-score)

The World Health Organization (WHO) defines osteoporosis as a T-score less than −2.5. A less severe form is osteopenia in which the T-score is −1.5 to −2.5.

Treatment includes weightbearing exercise to stimulate bone formation, dietary modification or supplementation with vitamin D and Ca, advice to expose skin to sunlight to generate more vitamin D, oestrogen supplementation (HRT increases risk of breast or uterine cancer) and pharmacological inhibition of osteoclasts using bisphosphonates.

Osteomalacia and rickets

These are qualitative defects in bone mineralisation. Rickets is the juvenile form, osteomalacia is the adult form. The result is painful microscopic stress fractures in long bones (known as Looser's zones or milkman's fractures); bowing of the long bones, especially the tibiae; vertebral collapse (codfish vertebrae); enlarged costochondral junctions (rachitic rosary); and retarded growth and short stature in children.

There are many causes but the commonest are:
- inherited defects in the hydroxylation of vitamin D;
- excessive loss of phosphate from the kidneys;
- lack of sunlight exposure in immigrant populations;
- dietary insufficiency.

Paget's disease

This is a condition usually seen in elderly patients whereby the normal interaction of osteoclasts and osteoblasts is lost. This results in excessive bone resorption by osteoclasts followed by disordered laying down of poor quality bone by osteoblasts. The result is coarse, weak bones, which may bow or bend and are often painful. Treatment is with bisphosphonates, which inhibit osteoclasts.

Osteopetrosis

This rare genetic condition, literally translated as stone bones, is due to failure of osteoclasts. Patients are unable to remodel bone in the normal way. This results in thick, hard, brittle bones that fracture easily.

③ Osteoarthritis

Figure 3.1 Weightbearing AP x-ray of an arthritic knee

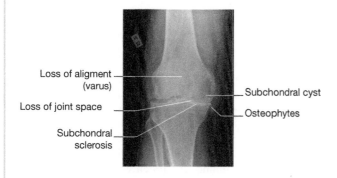

Loss of aligment (varus)

Loss of joint space

Subchondral sclerosis

Subchondral cyst

Osteophytes

Figure 3.2 Lateral x-ray of arthritic knee

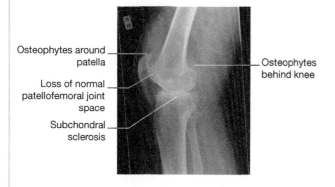

Osteophytes around patella

Loss of normal patellofemoral joint space

Subchondral sclerosis

Osteophytes behind knee

Figure 3.3 Severe OA of the right hip

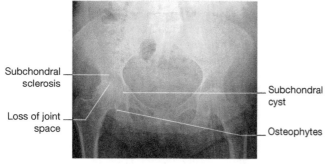

Subchondral sclerosis

Loss of joint space

Subchondral cyst

Osteophytes

Figure 3.4 Osteoarthritis Typically affects large synovial joints including hip, knee, first metatarsophalangeal joint of the foot, facet joints of the spine, shoulder and elbow. In the hand the interphalangeal joints and carpometacarpal joint at the base of the thumb may be affected

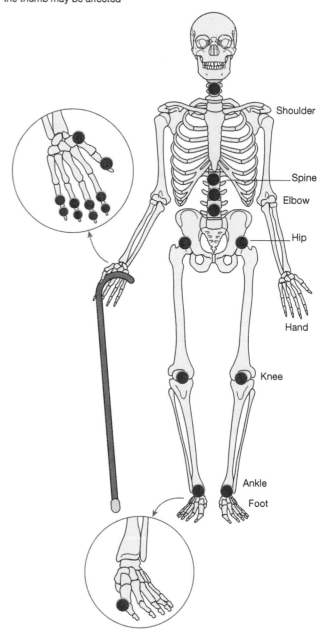

Shoulder

Spine

Elbow

Hip

Hand

Knee

Ankle
Foot

Trauma and Orthopaedics at a Glance, First Edition. Henry Willmott.
© 2016 John Wiley & Sons, Ltd. Published 2016 by John Wiley & Sons, Ltd. Companion website: www.ataglanceseries.com/TandO

Background

Osteoarthritis (OA) is the commonest condition encountered in elective orthopaedics. It is a non-inflammatory process and can affect all synovial joints, most frequently the knee. The commonest form of OA is primary, due to physiological 'wear-and-tear'. Secondary OA is caused by trauma – especially if the joint surface has been fractured and is no longer congruent – infection or congenital conditions.

The disease process starts with microscopic damage to the surface layers of articular cartilage. Paradoxically, the disease is self-perpetuating as attempts to repair microscopic damage result in increased levels of interleukins (especially IL-1) and activation of proteolytic enzymes that further degrade cartilage. As the disease progresses, the cartilage becomes softened (chondromalacia), fissured and frayed. Softening of the cartilage results in abnormal transmission of load to the subchondral bone, which results in mechanical failure of the bone in the form of microfractures. The bone attempts to heal these fractures by producing spurs of abnormal bone known as osteophytes, which can be seen on X-ray. Eventually underlying subchondral bone is exposed resulting in narrowing of the joint space on X-ray.

X-ray findings in OA (remember acronym LOSS)

- **L**oss of joint space (thinning of cartilage).
- **O**steophytes (attempts to repair underlying bone).
- **S**ubchondral sclerosis (hardening of bone in response to load).
- **S**ubchondral cysts (resulting from microfractures).

Clinical signs and symptoms

- Pain (worse on movement, disturbs sleep at night).
- Loss of movement ('stiffness' – inability to put socks on).
- Crepitus ('crunching').
- Instability ('giving way' due to loss of normal joint mechanics).

Diagnosis

- History & Examination – ask about previous trauma or infection, elicit severity of pain, including disturbance of sleep. Ask about limitation of function and work. Measure range of movement and note crepitus or instability. Comment on surrounding joints.
- X-rays – remember LOSS.
- MRI – helpful in early cases as cartilage is well visualised on MRI.
- CT – helpful in gross joint destruction to elicit where bone is damaged, but cartilage itself not visualised.
- Arthroscopy – not a primary diagnostic tool but useful for staging severity and treating limited areas of cartilage damage (see below).

Staging the severity of OA

The focus should be on the severity of the patient's symptoms. Surprisingly, there is a poor correlation with the degree of OA and the severity of symptoms. It is not unusual for a young patient with apparently very mild OA of the patellofemoral joint to be in a lot of pain, whereas an elderly patient with gross bone-on-bone OA is stoically carrying on! Perception of severity of symptoms is a combination of patient expectation and functional demands.

A more quantitative assessment method is **Outerbridge Staging**, used when viewing OA through an arthroscope:

- Grade 0 – normal
- Grade I – cartilage softening (chondromalacia)
- Grade II – partial-thickness defect with surface fissures
- Grade III – fissures extending down to subchondral bone
- Grade IV – exposed subchondral bone

Treatment

Conservative treatment should be tried at first:

- **Weight loss** – to reduce the load across the joint.
- **Activity modification** – avoidance of high-impact sports, modifying work duties, using a stick.
- **Physiotherapy** – to maintain the strength of muscles across the joint and maintain the range of movement. Proprioceptive exercises also help to reduce symptomatic instability.
- **Pharmacological treatment** – NSAIDS (non-steroidal anti-inflammatory drugs), simple analgesia, opiates.
- **Glucosamine** – the evidence that this reduces the pain of arthritis is limited, but it has few side-effects and is effective in some cases.

Surgical treatment is indicated if these have failed:

- **Injections** – steroid and local anaesthetic can be injected into arthritic joints. Although this may afford short-term relief from pain, the evidence for a long-lasting effect is poor. An alternative is to inject hyaluronic acid or synthetic derivatives thereof. This complex molecule is found naturally in synovial fluid and aids in lubrication. There are a number of hyaluronic acid-based products on the market but there is little evidence for their efficacy and some concern about potential side-effects. Their use is not widely recommended.
- **Arthroscopic intervention** – there is mounting evidence that arthroscopic washout of arthritic joints has no long-lasting effects. However, in young patients with a discrete lesion in the cartilage and no generalised OA, after trauma for example, the lesion can be treated arthroscopically. Options include microfracture, where the base of the lesion is drilled to stimulate bleeding and the formation of a fibrin clot to fill the defect; mosaicplasty, the transplant of healthy cartilage from one part of the joint to another; or implantation of cultured chondrocytes. Chondrocyte implantation is still in the developmental stages but initial results look promising.
- **Osteotomy** – in patients with arthritis affecting just the medial half of the knee and an associated varus deformity, the axis of the limb can be realigned by means of an osteotomy of the tibia. This transfers load away from the diseased area of cartilage. Although not curing the arthritis, it reduces pain.
- **Arthroplasty** (joint replacement) – the gold standard and most predictable way of treating OA. Most joints can now be replaced and this is discussed in the relevant chapters.
- **Arthrodesis** (fusion of the joint) – although a rather old-fashioned way of treating arthritis, this often represents a good option for failed arthroplasty, arthritis due to infection or treatment of small joints, in the hand or foot for example, where stability is more important than movement.

4 Rheumatoid arthritis

Figure 4.1 Manifestations of rheumatoid arthritis

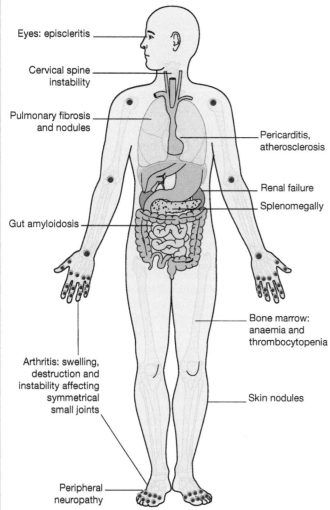

Eyes: episcleritis

Cervical spine instability

Pulmonary fibrosis and nodules

Pericarditis, atherosclerosis

Renal failure

Splenomegally

Gut amyloidosis

Bone marrow: anaemia and thrombocytopenia

Arthritis: swelling, destruction and instability affecting symmetrical small joints

Skin nodules

Peripheral neuropathy

Figure 4.2 A synovial joint Showing effusion, enlarged synovial lining, which invades the joint and is called pannus, erosions of bone and cartilage, attenuation of ligaments and joint instability

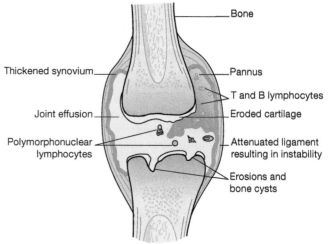

Thickened synovium

Joint effusion

Polymorphonuclear lymphocytes

Bone

Pannus

T and B lymphocytes

Eroded cartilage

Attenuated ligament resulting in instability

Erosions and bone cysts

Figure 4.3 X-ray of a rheumatoid hand

Note the ulnar drift of the fingers, subluxation of the metacarpophalangeal joints, z-deformity of the thumb, patchy osteoporosis and erosions around the joints

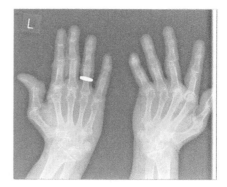

Trauma and Orthopaedics at a Glance, First Edition. Henry Willmott.
© 2016 John Wiley & Sons, Ltd. Published 2016 by John Wiley & Sons, Ltd. Companion website: www.ataglanceseries.com/TandO

Background

Rheumatoid arthritis (RA) is the commonest form of inflammatory arthritis. It affects 1% of the population, and is twice as common in women than in men. It is a multisystem autoimmune disease with a strong genetic component. The aetiology is not clear but theories exist citing environmental toxins or an infectious component combined with a genetic predisposition.

The underlying pathophysiology is a T-cell-driven autoimmune response in which complexes of antibodies are deposited within tissues.

In contrast to OA, RA has multisystemic manifestations affecting:

- **Synovial joints and associated tendons and ligaments** – multiple small joints are affected in a symmetrical distribution.
- **Skin** – deposition of immune complexes causes rheumatoid nodules, mainly on extensor surfaces.
- **Eyes** – episcleritis or keratoconjunctivitis sicca (dry eyes).
- **Cardiovascular and bronchopulmonary systems** – increased risk of atherosclerosis, pericarditis and rheumatoid nodules in the lungs.
- **Spleen and immune system** – Felty's syndrome is the combination of RA, splenomegaly and neutropenia.
- **Blood** – haematological manifestations include autoimmune anaemia and increased risk of lymphoma.
- **Kidneys** – deposits within the kidney cause renal impairment; amyloidosis may occur.
- **Nervous system** – peripheral neuropathy can occur, but more common is compression of nerves due to adjacent joint involvement, including carpal tunnel syndrome, cubital tunnel syndrome and compression of cervical nerves or spinal cord due to subluxation of the atlanto-axial joint in the neck.

Diagnosis

Certain diagnostic criteria have been developed in order to diagnose RA. Although there is some variability between the many and often complex sets of criteria, the common points are:

- Two or more swollen joints.
- Morning stiffness lasting more than an hour for at least six weeks.
- Positive rheumatoid factor or autoantibodies – rheumatoid factor (RhF) is an IgM to IgG antibody present in 80% of people with RA (called seropositive RA), but also present in 2% of normal people).

The differential diagnosis is large, but includes:

- **Crystal arthropathies** – gout and pseudogout, differentiated by the presence of crystals in joint aspirate and predilection for big toe metatarsophalangeal joint (MTPJ) and knee.
- **OA** – different joint distribution, absence of morning stiffness and older patient.
- **Reactive arthritis or Reiter's syndrome** – 'can't see, can't pee, can't bend the knee'.
- **Ankylosing spondylitis** – affects the sacroiliac joints and spine causing stiffness and stooped gait, but can also have associated small joint polyarthropathy.

- **Psoriatic arthropathy** – check for skin plaques on extensor surfaces as well as family history. Joint symptoms sometimes precede skin lesions.
- **SLE** (systemic lupus erythematosus) – malar rash and anti-double-stranded DNA antibodies.

X-ray findings in RA

X-rays of the hands and feet are performed as part of the diagnostic work-up for RA. Any other affected joints should also be X-rayed. The characteristic findings are:

- **Periarticular erosions** – synovitis erodes bone causing the formation of cysts.
- **Periarticular osteopenia** – loss of bone density occurs as a result of disuse due to pain and secondary effects of steroids.
- **Soft-tissue swelling** – subtle widening of the joint space may be seen when synovitis is mild. Severe synovitis is seen as gross swelling around the joints.
- **Joint subluxation and malalignment** – as ligaments become dysfunctional the joints sublux and can even dislocate. This gives rise to the classic deformities seen in hands and feet.

Treatment

The mainstay of RA is medical. Over the last several years there have been huge improvements in this field. As a result the manifestations of uncontrolled RA have been drastically reduced.

Surgeons must work as part of a multidisciplinary team in the treatment of this complex disease. Medical treatment is mainly coordinated by rheumatologists. It is important to have an idea of the main categories of drugs used:

- **anti-inflammatories**: NSAIDs; steroids (systemic or joint injection);
- **disease modifying anti-rheumatic drugs** (DMARDs): methotrexate, sulfasalazine, hydroxychloroquine;
- **biologic – anti-TNFα**: etanercept, infliximab.
- **biologic – anti-IL1**: anakinra;
- **monocolonal antibodies**: rituximab.

The role of the orthopaedic surgeon is to address the secondary sequelae of periarticular RA. These include:

- **Instability** of joints due to ligament destruction – joint replacement, arthrodesis (fusion), soft-tissue procedures to restore stability.
- **Pain** due to instability and synovitis – address instability with reconstruction of ligaments or fusion of the joint, perform synovectomy to remove pain-generating inflamed synovial tissue.
- **Nerve compression** – synovectomy and decompression of peripheral nerves, especially median nerve at wrist, ulnar nerve at elbow.
- **Tendon dysfunction** due to erosion by inflamed synovium – reconstruction of affected tendons, usually by performing tendon transfer (repositioning a nearby healthy tendon to reproduce the function of the dysfunctional tendon).

These topics are addressed in greater detail in the relevant chapters.

Imaging in orthopaedics: X-rays

Figure 5.1 X-ray generation

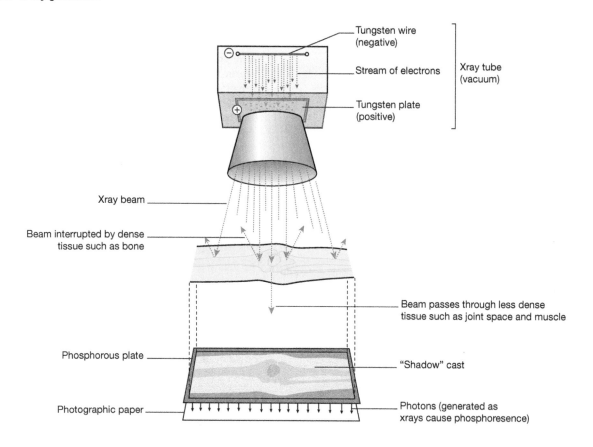

Tungsten wire (negative)

Stream of electrons

Xray tube (vacuum)

Tungsten plate (positive)

Xray beam

Beam interrupted by dense tissue such as bone

Beam passes through less dense tissue such as joint space and muscle

Phosphorous plate

"Shadow" cast

Photographic paper

Photons (generated as xrays cause phosphoresence)

Figure 5.2 X-ray of wrist
AP and lateral. An x-ray is a 2-dimensional representation of a 3-dimensional structure. Here there is a dislocation of the carpus which can only be properly appreciated on the lateral view. Always obtain orthogonal images

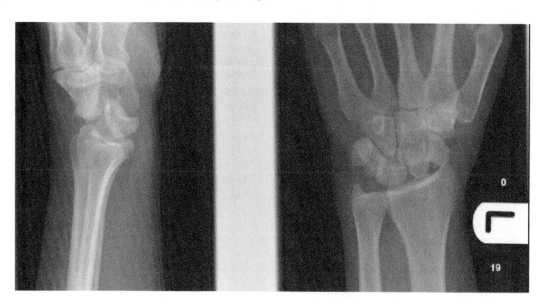

Trauma and Orthopaedics at a Glance, First Edition. Henry Willmott.
© 2016 John Wiley & Sons, Ltd. Published 2016 by John Wiley & Sons, Ltd. Companion website: www.ataglanceseries.com/TandO

X-ray generation and radiographs

Radiographs, also known as roentgenograms or X-rays are the most widely used imaging modality in orthopaedics. Discovered in 1895 by German physicist Wilhelm Röntgen, the first image of a human body part was of Röntgen's wife's hand.

The X-ray beam is generated by the X-ray tube. This is composed of a metal wire that is heated by a high-voltage electric current. The wire emits electrons, which strike a positively charged tungsten plate. Collisions between electrons and tungsten molecules generate X-rays.

X-rays are part of the electromagnetic spectrum, between UV and gamma rays. It is ionising radiation and can damage cellular DNA. This can cause mutations and cancer. The risk of cancer is low and depends on the age of the patient, the body part being imaged and the amount of X-rays to which the patient (or clinician) is exposed. A chest X-ray is the equivalent of 10 days' background radiation, whereas a cervical-spine X-ray is equivalent to 6 months' worth. Although the risk is small, it should always be considered when requesting X-ray investigations, especially if the patient is pregnant.

Radiographs are produced by placing a body part between the tube and the receiving plate. Traditionally, this was a phosphorus-coated sheet of glass underneath which was a sheet of photographic film. As the X-rays struck the phosphorus, photons were generated, which were detected by the photographic film. This was then developed in a dark room. Modern technology has superseded this last step, and the photons are now detected by electronic means, instantly producing a digital image.

Tissue that is radiodense, such as bone, block or attenuate the beam more than tissues that are less radiodense, such as fat or muscle. This property means that a 'shadow' is cast on the plate.

An appreciation of the 'shadow' analogy by which radiographs are produced will help you interpret the images. Imagine a desk lamp shining onto a wall. If you hold your hand close to the light source, the image produced is large. A hand close to the wall will produce a smaller image. Similarly, opaque material, such as this book, will produce a shadow that is darker than that produced by more translucent material, such as a thin sheet of paper.

Radiographs of the human body are exactly the same, although the image is in negative – more radiodense structures produce a very white image, less radiodense structures are darker grey. Air is the least radiodense material in the human body and attenuates virtually no X-rays, thus producing a very black image. Fat and muscle are of intermediate radiodensity. Furthermore, structures close to the X-ray tube will appear larger than those further away.

Radiographic terminology

Various terms are used to describe radiographs and there are some that you should be familiar with:
- **P-A or A-P** – this signifies the direction of the X-ray beam, either from posterior to anterior, or anterior to posterior. The implication of this is that anterior structures will appear more magnified on the A-P and vice versa.
- **Lateral** – a 'side' view relative to the anatomical position. The combination of two perpendicular (orthogonal) images is vital when imaging a bone or joint in order to appreciate the three-dimensional nature of the body part.
- **Frog-leg lateral** – a way of obtaining lateral images of both hips in children. The child is lain on his or her back with hips flexed and abducted, like a frog.
- **Skyline** – a method of imaging the underside of the patella and its relationship to the trochlear groove of the distal femur. The knee is maximally flexed and the X-ray beam directed longitudinally underneath the patella.
- **Mortice** – a view used when imaging the ankle, demonstrating the talus centrally placed between the medial and lateral malleoli. It differs from a true A-P because the leg is internally rotated by 15° to prevent overlap of the bones.
- **Axillary** – when imaging the shoulder, the plate can be placed in the patient's axilla, and the beam fired from above the patient's head This demonstrates the relationship of the humeral head to the glenoid and demonstrates if it is dislocated anteriorly or posteriorly. They can be hard to interpret, but reliably demonstrate a dislocation.
- **Scapular-Y** – another shoulder view (there are many more!), whereby the beam is fired horizontally in the plane of the scapula, to demonstrate the humeral head overlying the glenoid. It is another way of demonstrating a dislocation.
- **Image intensifier (I.I.), fluoroscopy** – images in theatre are produced by an image intensifier. This is a machine composed of a 'C-arm' with a tube at one end and a receiving plate at the other, linked to a television screen. The images are produced in real time and in exactly the same way as traditional radiographs, but are inverted – bone is black, air is white.
- **Red dot** – in the past, when radiographs were produced on photographic film, the radiographer would stick a small red sticker on any images that they felt were abnormal. Now most images are digital and the stickers are redundant. However, astute radiographers will still write the words on abnormal images. Chances are that they have seen many more radiographs than you, so take note!

Basics of radiograph interpretation

This topic is covered in more detail in Chapter 48, but when looking at a radiograph, there are a few key points you should check and if presenting, comment on:
- **Patient name and number** – usually displayed at the top right of the image.
- **Date and time** at which the image was generated – it is easy to mistakenly open an older image when using digital archives.
- **The body part** being imaged.
- **The view** – and if you have only been shown either an A-P or a lateral, ask for an orthogonal view – you *must* have both in order to evaluate the 3D configuration.
- **The adequacy** of the view – is the whole bone or joint included?
- **The abnormality** – it may not always be apparent, but if you can clearly see a fracture or arthritis, say so! If it is not obvious, trace the cortices of each bone looking for a breach.
- **Associated features** such as a joint effusion, soft tissue swelling, the presence of plaster cast, etc.

6 Imaging in orthopaedics: other modalities

Figure 6.1   CT

Patient moved sequentially
through scanner

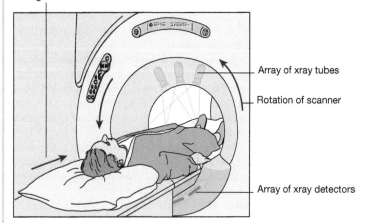

Array of xray tubes

Rotation of scanner

Array of xray detectors

Figure 6.2   Cross-sectional imaging terminology

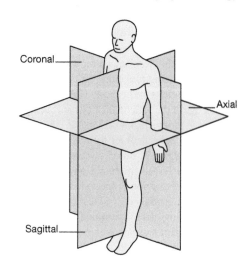

Coronal

Axial

Sagittal

Figure 6.3   MRI

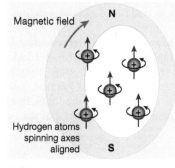

Magnetic field

N

Hydrogen atoms
spinning axes
aligned

S

(a) Strong magnet aligns the axes of
spinning hydrogen atoms

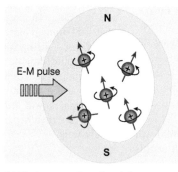

N

E-M pulse

S

(b) Electromagnetic pulse deflects
all axes

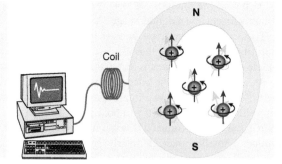

Coil

N

S

(c) When pulse stops, coil connected
to computer detects rate of return
to resting state in different tissues

Figure 6.4   Ultrasound

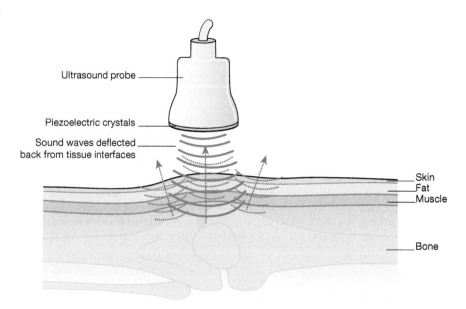

Ultrasound probe

Piezoelectric crystals

Sound waves deflected
back from tissue interfaces

Skin
Fat
Muscle

Bone

Trauma and Orthopaedics at a Glance, First Edition. Henry Willmott.
© 2016 John Wiley & Sons, Ltd. Published 2016 by John Wiley & Sons, Ltd. Companion website: www.ataglanceseries.com/TandO

Computed tomography (CT)

An inherent weakness of plain X-ray radiography is that a three-dimensional structure is represented by a two-dimensional image. Although two orthogonal images go some way to addressing this, X-rays of complex structures such as the spine and pelvis can be difficult to interpret. Computed tomography addresses this issue.

The scanner produces multiple cross-sectional X-ray images, which are reformatted by a computer to produce reconstructions in three dimensions. The images are produced by the *CT gantry*, which is an X-ray tube positioned opposite an array of detectors. The tube rotates around the patient, generating one *slice*. The patient is sequentially moved through the gantry, so generating multiple slices. More modern *spiral CT* scanners decrease the time needed to scan by moving the patient continually during image acquisition.

The computer can generate reconstructions in any plane, but the standard is three sequences:
- **Axial** – horizontal slices perpendicular to the axis of the body.
- **Sagittal** – longitudinal slices from anterior to posterior (derived from the Latin for 'arrow'; think of Harold in 1066).
- **Coronal** – longitudinal slices from left to right (derived from the Latin for 'crown').

It is also possible to generate 3D renderings.

CT uses X-rays and is therefore better at visualising bone than soft tissue. Imaging of soft tissues, particularly the more vascular organs, can be improved by using IV contrast, although this is nephrotoxic. The radiation dose is considerably larger than that of plain X-rays.

Magnetic resonance imaging (MRI)

The soft tissues of the body contain large amounts of water. Water contains two hydrogen atoms, each composed of a negatively charged electron orbiting around a positive nucleus. The spin of the electron generates a tiny magnetic field. An MRI scanner can detect fluctuations within this field to determine the density of water in tissue.

The scanner is composed of a large *magnet* and a *detector coil*. The magnet aligns the axis of spin and therefore the magnetic fields of all the hydrogen molecules within the body. An electromagnetic pulse is then applied at 90° to the magnetic field. This momentarily deflects the alignment of the hydrogen molecules.

This 'wobble' and the time taken for it to return to a steady state are detected by the detector coil. Complex computer algorithms generate 3D reconstructions in the three standard planes.

Modifications of the electromagnetic pulse and the detection algorithm allow the generation of different *sequences*, which focus on water, fat or oedema. The most commonly used sequences are listed:
- T1 – shows fat as white, water as dark. Useful for looking at tendons, ligaments and complex soft-tissue structures.
- T2 – shows water as white, fat as dark. Useful for looking at disc prolapses in the spine as the CSF in the dural sac is white and the disc annulus is dark.
- STIR – stands for *short-tau inversion recovery* and shows oedema and inflammation as bright white with normal tissue very dark. Shows bone bruising, torn ligaments and menisci.

Although MRI does not expose the patient to radiation, the very strong magnet in the scanner can be hazardous if metal objects are inadvertently taken into the scanning room. Scissors, oxygen cylinders and even beds can become lethal projectiles. Intubated patients who are connected to a mechanical ventilator present a management challenge. Patients with pacemakers or metallic heart valves cannot go into the scanner. Obese patients may be too large to fit into the scanner and many patients find it claustrophobic.

Ultrasound (US)

Ultrasound uses the deflection of sound waves to generate images. The ultrasound probe is composed of piezoelectric crystals that emit an ultrasonic sound wave when a current is passed across them. The sound wave bounces off the boundary between tissues of different densities and is detected by the probe as an echo.

More advanced scanners can detect the flow of fluid within vessels, detected by means of the Doppler effect.

The images produced are two-dimensional and their creation is very user-dependent. Interpretation of saved images after they have been obtained is difficult.

Nevertheless, this modality allows dynamic screening of soft tissues such as tendon, muscle, ligament and the soft organs of the abdominal cavity. In experienced hands it is quick and can be very useful in the context of trauma to determine if there is free fluid or blood within the abdominal cavity (this application is known as FAST scanning – *focused abdominal sonography for trauma*).

Choice of imaging modality

	Pros	Cons	Suggested use
X-ray	Cheap, easily available, mobile images in A&E if unstable patient	Radiation (low dose), poor imaging of complex structures, poor demonstration of soft tissue	Arthritis, fractures, chest
CT	Available in most hospitals, spiral CT is quick, 3D imaging of complex structures	High dose of radiation, patient needs to be transported to scanner, limited imaging of ligament/tendon/disc	Complex fractures (spine, tibial plateau, pilon, pelvis)
MRI	Excellent imaging of soft tissues, shows oedema and inflammation, no radiation	Poor resolution of bone, slow, patient needs to be transported to scanner, claustrophobia, weight limit, magnet precludes pacemakers	Spinal disc prolapse, ligamentous or meniscal injury, osteomyelitis
US	Dynamic, may be interventional, no radiation	Difficult to master and interpret, operator dependent, poor at demonstrating bone	Tendon rupture, foreign bodies, 'FAST' in trauma

7 Infection

Figure 7.1 Septic arthritis Patients present with severe pain which is exacerbated by any movement of the affected joint. Left untreated, they may become septic, exhibiting fever, tachycardia, hypertension and shock

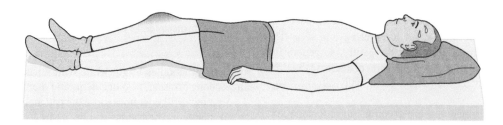

Figure 7.2 Acute haematogenous osteomyelitis is the commonest cause of osteomyelitis and septic arthritis in children

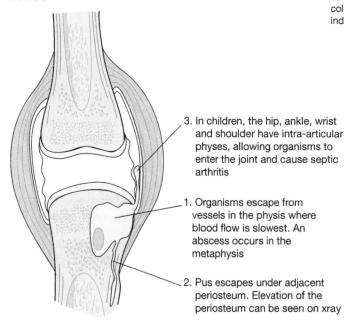

3. In children, the hip, ankle, wrist and shoulder have intra-articular physes, allowing organisms to enter the joint and cause septic arthritis

1. Organisms escape from vessels in the physis where blood flow is slowest. An abscess occurs in the metaphysis

2. Pus escapes under adjacent periosteum. Elevation of the periosteum can be seen on xray

Figure 7.3 Discitis This T2 weighted MRI of the lumbar spine shows increased signal (bright) within the disc of L2–3 with expansion into the surrounding tissues. This is typical of discitis. There is no abscess or collection at this stage, so surgical decompression would not be indicated

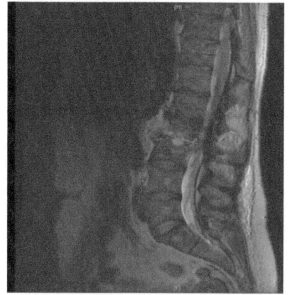

Figure 7.4a Gram staining Gram positive organisms appear blue on gram stain, staphlococcus aureus are gram positive cocci in clusters and look like bunches of grapes

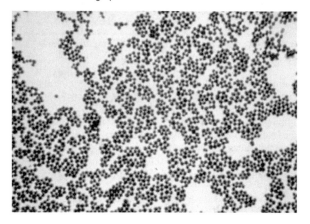

Figure 7.4b Gram negative organisms appear red, these gram negative rods are pseudomonas

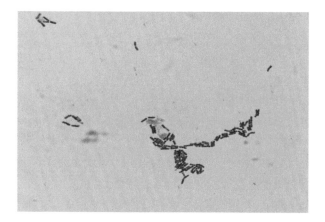

Infection of joint replacements is covered separately in Chapters 20 and 21.

Osteomyelitis

Infection of bone is known as osteomyelitis. It can occur either because of direct exposure of the bone to a dirty environment, after an open fracture for example, or more commonly, due to haematogenous spread of blood-borne organisms. This is known as *acute haematogenous osteomyelitis* (AHO).

AHO is much more common in children, although some adults are susceptible, especially those with immunocompromise, diabetes, renal disease, sickle-cell disease or IV drug users. The causative bacteraemia can occur with an infection elsewhere or after vigorous tooth brushing!

The commonest site of bone infection is where blood flow is slowest. This is at the growth plate in the metaphyses of bones. Slow flow allows bacteria to exit the vessels and form a subperiosteal abscess. Some joints, namely the shoulder, wrist, hip and ankle, have a capsule that extends far enough to incorporate the adjacent growth plates. Should osteomyelitis start in one of these growth plates, then bacteria can escape into the joint and cause secondary septic arthritis.

The diagnosis of osteomyelitis is often delayed in children. Any child with unexplained pain and signs of infection should be investigated for osteomyelitis. Investigations should include plain X-ray, which may demonstrate periosteal elevation and soft-tissue swelling. In advanced cases a radiolucent area may be seen. Blood should include C-reactive protein (CRP; most sensitive, rises fastest), erythrocyte sedimentation rate (ESR; less sensitive, takes 3 days to rise), white cell count (WCC; may be normal) and blood cultures (taken ideally before antibiotics are started). An MRI may demonstrate abscess formation and this is an indication for surgery. If no abscess is found, antibiotics are the mainstay of treatment.

Septic arthritis

Infection within the joint capsule may occur in children due to haematogenous spread of organisms, direct inoculation of a joint due to trauma, or spread of adjacent osteomyelitis. In adults direct inoculation or post-surgical infections are more common.

Septic arthritis is a surgical emergency. Bacteria produce enzymes that rapidly destroy cartilage causing devastating secondary arthritis. Patients can also become septic and shocked.

It is vital to have a high index of suspicion. Any child who is limping, unable to bear weight or has an unexplained fever should be investigated. A suddenly swollen painful joint in an adult is highly suspicious.

Examination may reveal a joint effusion. The patient will be unwilling to move the joint. Look for warmth, erythema or skin changes as well as any evidence of penetrating wounds. In children perform a systematic examination to exclude other causes of infection.

Investigations should include WCC, which may be normal initially; CRP and ESR, which are very sensitive but not specific; blood cultures, which are positive in around 30%; and plain X-rays, which may demonstrate an effusion or adjacent osteomyelitis. The most sensitive and specific investigation is a joint aspiration. Children generally need this performing under anaesthetic, but most adult joints can be aspirated in A&E. See Chapter 52 for details. Send specimens for microscopy, culture and sensitivity (MC&S) and also ask the lab to check for crystals. **Never aspirate a joint-replacement in A&E or on the ward!** The risk of accidentally introducing infection is high and it should only be done in theatre!

Microscopy of the aspirate may reveal visible organisms, in which case the diagnosis is clear. The white cell count of the aspirate is helpful: >50,000 cells/mL and >75% neutrophils is typical of septic arthritis. Culture results take 3–4 days.

Treatment is irrigation of the affected joint, either arthroscopic or open, combined with several weeks of antibiotics.

Soft-tissue infections

An abscess forms when bacteria become walled-off from the immune system by granulation tissue. Treatment is surgical incision and drainage of pus. The wound should be left open or packed to prevent the abscess re-forming.

Necrotising fasciitis is an uncommon but serious condition of rapidly spreading infection along fascial planes, often with limited skin signs. It is more common in diabetics, IV drug users and alcoholics. Patients appear much more unwell than would be expected, often with very high temperatures. Initial findings may be unimpressive with localised pain and induration. Left untreated bullae, blisters and gangrene develop. Production of toxins causes overwhelming septic shock, which is often fatal. Aggressive debridement and high-dose antibiotics are indicated.

Discitis

Infection can form within intervertebral discs. This is a cause of chronic back pain, often in the elderly or immunosuppressed. The poor blood supply of the disc makes it hard to deliver antibiotics to the area. Long courses of antibiotics are needed. If an abscess forms, it can put pressure on the spinal cord or nerves and require surgical decompression. Tuberculosis infection, commoner in developing countries, causes vertebral bone destruction, leading to instability and deformity.

Common organisms

Septic arthritis and osteomyelitis	
Neonates	Group B streptococci, *Staphylococcus aureus*
Children <4 years	*Staph. aureus*, *Streptococcus pneumoniae*, Group A streptococci, *Haemophilus influenzae*
Children >4 year and adults	*Staph. aureus*
Young adults/adolescents	*Neisseria gonorrhoeae*
Immunosuppressed/IV drug users	Tuberculosis, fungi, *Pseudomonas aeruginosa*
Sickle-cell disease	*Staph. aureus*, *Salmonella*

Soft-tissue infections	
General	*Staph. aureus*, streptococci, MRSA
Shoe puncture	*Pseudomonas aeruginosa*
Necrotising fasciitis	*Streptococcus pyogenes*, mixed
Gas gangrene	*Clostridium perfringens*
Animal and human bites	*Pasteurella multocida*, *Eikenella corrodens*

8 Clinical anatomy of the upper limb

Figure 8.1 Posterior and anterior views of the left scapula

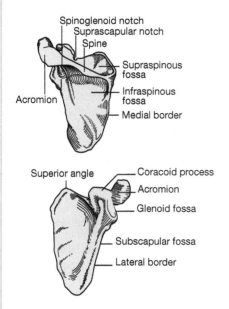

Spinoglenoid notch
Suprascapular notch
Spine
Supraspinous fossa
Infraspinous fossa
Acromion
Medial border

Superior angle
Coracoid process
Acromion
Glenoid fossa
Subscapular fossa
Lateral border

Figure 8.2 Anterior and posterior views of the left humerus

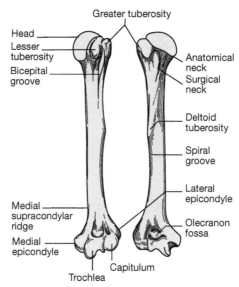

Greater tuberosity
Head
Lesser tuberosity
Bicepital groove
Anatomical neck
Surgical neck
Deltoid tuberosity
Spiral groove
Lateral epicondyle
Medial supracondylar ridge
Olecranon fossa
Medial epicondyle
Capitulum
Trochlea

Figure 8.3 The left radius and ulna in (a) supination and (b) pronation

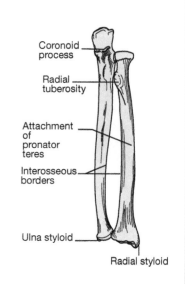

Coronoid process
Radial tuberosity
Attachment of pronator teres
Interosseous borders
Ulna styloid
Radial styloid

Figure 8.4 The skeleton of the left hand, holding a cross-section through the carpal tunnel

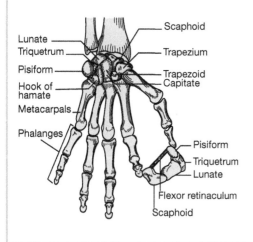

Lunate
Triquetrum
Pisiform
Hook of hamate
Metacarpals
Phalanges
Scaphoid
Trapezium
Trapezoid
Capitate
Pisiform
Triquetrum
Lunate
Flexor retinaculum
Scaphoid

Figure 8.5 The main blood vessels and nerves of the front of the arm

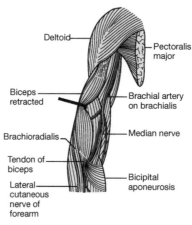

Deltoid
Pectoralis major
Biceps retracted
Brachial artery on brachialis
Brachioradialis
Median nerve
Tendon of biceps
Bicipital aponeurosis
Lateral cutaneous nerve of forearm

Figure 8.6 The major nerves in the back of the arm

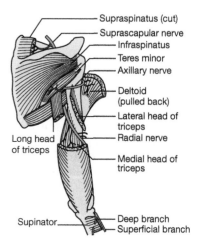

Supraspinatus (cut)
Suprascapular nerve
Infraspinatus
Teres minor
Axillary nerve
Deltoid (pulled back)
Lateral head of triceps
Radial nerve
Long head of triceps
Medial head of triceps
Supinator
Deep branch
Superficial branch

Trauma and Orthopaedics at a Glance, First Edition. Henry Willmott.
© 2016 John Wiley & Sons, Ltd. Published 2016 by John Wiley & Sons, Ltd. Companion website: www.ataglanceseries.com/TandO

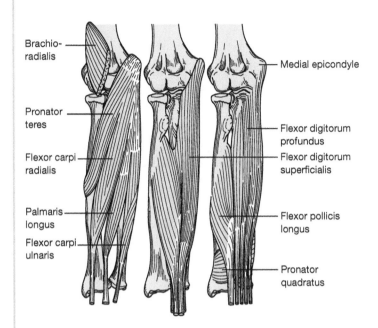

Figure 8.7 The superficial, intermediate and deep layers of muscles in the anterior (flexor) compartment of the right forearm

Brachio-radialis

Pronator teres

Flexor carpi radialis

Palmaris longus

Flexor carpi ulnaris

Medial epicondyle

Flexor digitorum profundus

Flexor digitorum superficialis

Flexor pollicis longus

Pronator quadratus

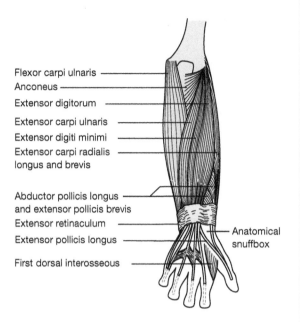

Figure 8.8 The muscles of the superficial and deep layers of the posterior (extensor) compartment of the forearm

Flexor carpi ulnaris

Anconeus

Extensor digitorum

Extensor carpi ulnaris

Extensor digiti minimi

Extensor carpi radialis longus and brevis

Abductor pollicis longus and extensor pollicis brevis

Extensor retinaculum

Extensor pollicis longus

First dorsal interosseous

Anatomical snuffbox

The shoulder

The humerus articulates with the glenoid, which is a protuberance arising from the scapula. The joint is very shallow so has a good range of movement but is prone to dislocation. The humeral head is stabilised by a cartilage lip called the labrum, strong ligaments and a hood of muscles called the rotator cuff. Draped over the shoulder joint is the deltoid, which is a large muscle that acts to abduct the arm. The deltoid is supplied by the axillary nerve, which loops around the neck of the humerus. If the shoulder is dislocated or the proximal humerus is fractured, the axillary nerve can be injured, resulting in wasting of the deltoid and numbness of the overlying skin.

The scapula is connected to the thorax by the clavicle, which acts like a strut. At each end of the clavicle is a joint: the sternoclavicular joint medially and the acromioclavicular joint laterally. These joints can be disrupted or dislocated in a fall.

Beneath the clavicle is a network of nerves called the brachial plexus, as well as the subclavian artery, vein and the apex of the lung. All these structures are vulnerable if the clavicle is fractured.

The humerus

At the proximal end of the humerus is the head, below which is the anatomical neck. This is of little clinical relevance. The surgical neck is slightly more distal and as the bone narrows here, there is a weak point prone to fracture.

The greater tuberosity is a bony prominence that is the insertion of the supraspinatus muscle, responsible for abducting the arm.

Along the posterior edge of the humerus is the spiral groove where the radial nerve runs close to bone. The nerve can be injured if the humerus is fractured, resulting in wrist drop and numbness in the first dorsal webspace of the hand.

Posterior to the humerus is the triceps muscle, innervated by the radial nerve and producing extension at the elbow. The triceps muscle can be split in the line of its fibres to provide access to the humerus for surgical fixation.

Anteriorly lies the coracobrachialis, brachialis and biceps muscles, which between them extend the arm at the elbow, flex the elbow and supinate the forearm. Beneath the biceps lie the brachial artery and median nerves.

The elbow

The distal humerus has a bulbous protuberance called the coronoid, which articulates with the radial head. The radial head, stabilised by the annular ligament, rotates to produce pronation (palm down) and supination (palm up). Medially, the ulna articulates with a groove in the end of the humerus called the trochlea. The proximal ulna has a prominent olecranon, which provides insertion for the triceps tendon. Falling onto the elbow can fracture the olecranon, compromising the ability to extend the elbow.

The medial epicondyle provides insertion for all the flexors of the wrist. It is known as the common flexor origin. The lateral epicondyle is the insertion of the wrist extensors and is called the common extensor origin. Inflammation of the tendons here is called tennis elbow.

The forearm

On the anterior aspect of the forearm lie the wrist and finger flexors. They comprise pronator teres (which also pronates the forearm), flexor carpi radialis, palmaris longus, flexor carpi ulnaris and flexor digitorum superficialis. Deep to these are flexor digitorum profundus and flexor pollicis longus. They are all innervated by the medial nerve apart from flexor carpi ulnaris and half of flexor digitorum profundus, which are innervated by the ulnar nerve. The median nerve and radial and ulnar arteries run between the deep and superficial muscle groups.

On the posterior aspect of the forearm are the wrist and finger extensors comprising extensor digitorum, extensor digiti minimi, extensor carpi ulnaris, supinator, extensor pollicis longus and brevis and extensor digitorum indicis. They are all innervated by the radial nerve.

There is a third group of muscles called the 'mobile wad', which runs from the lateral aspect of the distal humerus down to the wrist. These are brachioradialis, extensor carpi radialis longus and extensor carpi radialis brevis. These are also innervated by the radial nerve. Beneath the mobile wad runs the sensory branch of the radial nerve. The interval between the mobile wad and the flexors is a convenient surgical approach to the distal radius, provided the nerve is protected.

The wrist

At the wrist the distal radius articulates with the carpal bones. These are arranged in two rows. The scaphoid, lunate, triquetrum and pisiform make the proximal row. The trapezium, trapezoid, capitate and hamate make the distal row. There is limited movement between the rows, which are stabilised by strong ligaments The scaphoid is the most frequently fractured carpal bone, which sometimes disrupts its blood supply resulting in non-union and avascular necrosis.

On the anterior ('palmar' or 'volar') side of the carpal bones is the carpal tunnel, the roof of which is the tough carpal ligament. The median nerve and nine tendons run through the tunnel. Swelling or inflammation may squeeze the nerve resulting in carpal tunnel syndrome.

The hand

The metacarpals articulate with the carpal bones. Distally the fingers are made up of three phalanges. The thumb has two phalanges. The extensor tendons are on the dorsal side, the flexor tendons are on the volar side.

The flexor tendons in the fingers have a complex structure. Flexor digitorum superficialis inserts into the base of the middle phalanx and flexes the proximal interphalangeal joint. Flexor digitorum profundus splits to pass around the flexor digitorum superficialis (FDS) tendon before inserting into the distal phalanx to flex the distal interphalangeal joint.

In order to keep the flexor tendons close to bone, there is a network of pulleys that form a sheath. If a wound on the volar side of the finger gets infected, the infection can travel up the sheath into the palm. The result is severe scarring in the sheath resulting in a stiff finger.

9 Clinical anatomy of the lower limb

Figure 9.1 The bony anatomy of the pelvis

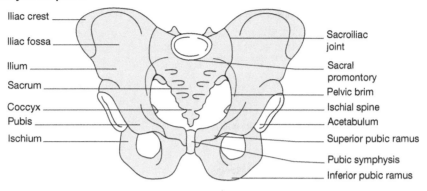

- Iliac crest
- Iliac fossa
- Ilium
- Sacrum
- Coccyx
- Pubis
- Ischium
- Sacroiliac joint
- Sacral promontory
- Pelvic brim
- Ischial spine
- Acetabulum
- Superior pubic ramus
- Pubic symphysis
- Inferior pubic ramus

Figure 9.2 The femur

- Piriformis fossa
- Nutrient foramina
- Greater trochanter
- Head
- Intertrochanteric line
- Lesser trochanter
- Trochlea
- Lateral condyle
- Medial condyle

Figure 9.3 The muscles of the front of the thigh. The femoral triangle is outlined

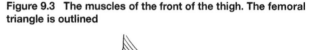

- Tensor fasciae latae
- Rectus femoris
- Vastus lateralis
- Iliotibial tract
- Patellar retinacula
- Iliacus
- Femoral triangle
- Inguinal ligament
- Psoas tendon
- Pectineus
- Adductor longus
- Gracilis
- Sartorius
- Vastus medialis
- Quadriceps tendon
- Patella tendon

Figure 9.4 Anterior view of the flexed right knee joint after division of the quadriceps and retraction of the patella

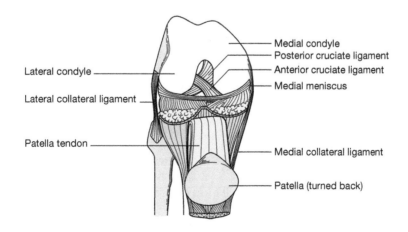

- Lateral condyle
- Lateral collateral ligament
- Patella tendon
- Medial condyle
- Posterior cruciate ligament
- Anterior cruciate ligament
- Medial meniscus
- Medial collateral ligament
- Patella (turned back)

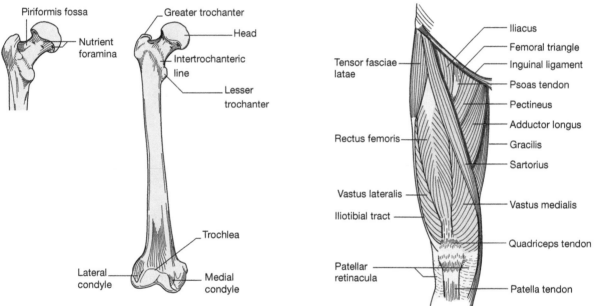

Trauma and Orthopaedics at a Glance, First Edition. Henry Willmott.
© 2016 John Wiley & Sons, Ltd. Published 2016 by John Wiley & Sons, Ltd. Companion website: www.ataglanceseries.com/TandO

Figure 9.5 The extensor (dorsiflexor) group of muscles

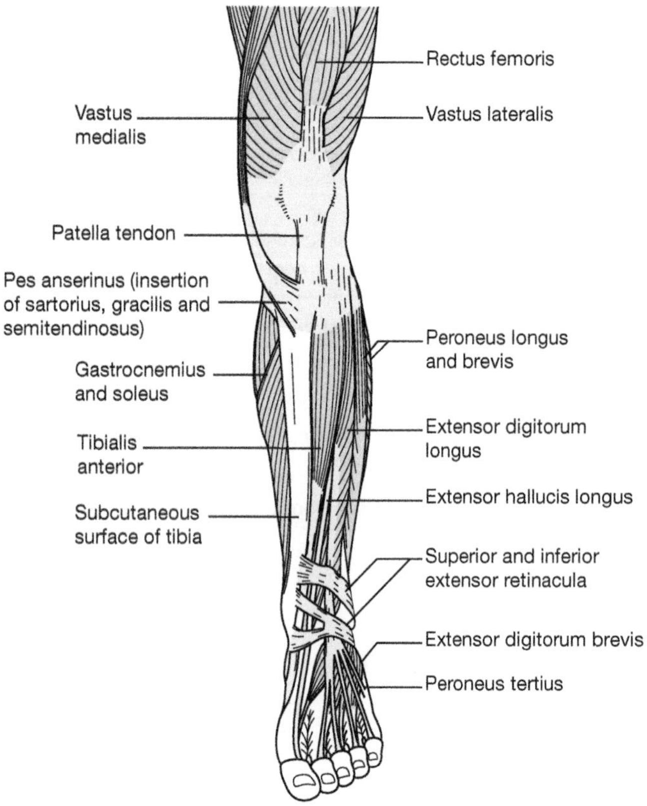

Rectus femoris
Vastus lateralis
Vastus medialis
Patella tendon
Pes anserinus (insertion of sartorius, gracilis and semitendinosus)
Gastrocnemius and soleus
Tibialis anterior
Subcutaneous surface of tibia
Peroneus longus and brevis
Extensor digitorum longus
Extensor hallucis longus
Superior and inferior extensor retinacula
Extensor digitorum brevis
Peroneus tertius

Figure 9.6 The lateral side of the leg and foot

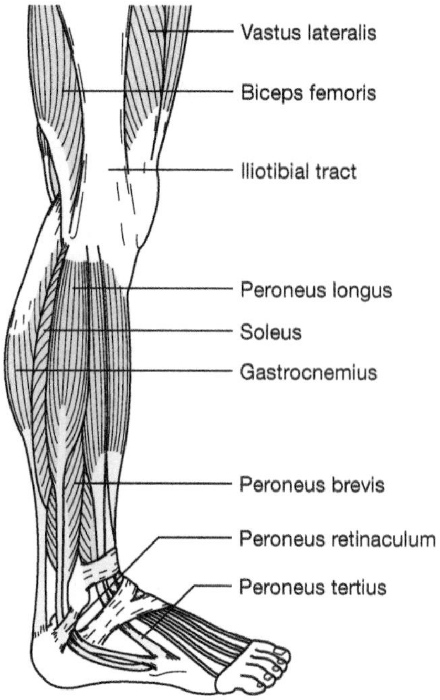

Vastus lateralis
Biceps femoris
Iliotibial tract
Peroneus longus
Soleus
Gastrocnemius
Peroneus brevis
Peroneus retinaculum
Peroneus tertius

Pelvis

The pelvis is composed of two innominate bones joined by the sacrum posteriorly. Each innominate bone is composed of three united bones: ilium, ischium and pubis. Closely related to the bones of the pelvis are the internal and external iliac arteries, a rich plexus of veins, the bladder, ureters, rectum, prostate and vagina. Fracture of the pelvis can result in massive haemorrhage or injury to the pelvic organs.

Hip

The hip is a ball-and-socket joint composed of the acetabulum and the femoral head. The acetabulum is deepened by a cartilaginous labrum (lip). The depth of the joint means that it is inherently stable.

The hip has a tough capsule that inserts into the intertrochanteric crest of the femur. At this level a ring of arteries sends blood vessels to the femoral head. The vessels are closely apposed to the femoral neck and can be injured if the femoral neck is fractured within the capsule, resulting in avascular necrosis of the femoral head.

Outside the capsule, the greater trochanter of the femur is a bony prominence that provides insertion for the gluteus medius and gluteus minimus. These are abductors of the hip. Injury to these muscles or the greater trochanter results in a Trendelenburg gait.

The lesser trochanter is a smaller prominence where the iliopsoas tendon inserts. This flexes the hip.

Posterior to the hip runs the sciatic nerve. The nerve can be injured during hip surgery or following a dislocation. This results in foot drop and numbness.

Thigh

The femur is surrounded by muscle. Anteriorly lies the quadriceps, which has four parts: vastus lateralis, vastus intermedius, vastus medialis and rectus femoris. This powerful muscle, innervated by the femoral nerve, extends the knee.

Posteriorly lie the hamstrings, semitendinosus, semimembranosus, and biceps femoris. These are innervated by branches of the sciatic nerve. The interval between the lateral edge of quadriceps and the posterior compartment provides convenient surgical access to the femoral shaft.

Medially lie the adductors, gracilis and sartorius. The femoral artery and vein run with this muscle group.

Surrounding the muscles of the thigh is a tough fascial layer called the fascia lata. Septa extend deep from the fascia to divide the three groups of muscles into separate compartments. Swelling of the muscles after trauma can increase the pressure within the compartments, resulting in compartment syndrome.

Knee

The knee is the articulation between the femur, tibia and patella. The two femoral condyles articulate with the tibial plateau. The space between the femoral condyles is known as the notch and houses the anterior and posterior cruciate ligaments. These prevent anterior and posterior subluxation of the tibia, respectively. Injury to the anterior cruciate ligament (ACL) is common in skiers and footballers. The result is instability when attempting twisting movements.

The patella is a sesamoid bone within the tendon of quadriceps. It helps the quadriceps to function efficiently and glide smoothly across the front of the femur. It sits in a groove called the trochlea.

Either side of the knee are the medial and lateral collateral ligaments. These may be sprained or torn if violent varus or valgus force is applied to the knee.

Lying within the joint space between the femur and tibia are two fibrocartilaginous structures called the medial and lateral menisci. They act as shock absorbers and help distribute force across the joint surfaces. The lateral meniscus is larger and more mobile, whereas the medial meniscus is fixed and is smaller. The menisci can be torn, resulting in painful clicking and sometimes locking of the knee.

Leg

The tibia is triangular in cross-section with a prominent anteromedial border just beneath the skin. Fracture of the tibia may result in the bone penetrating the skin, called an open fracture.

There are three groups of muscles:
• Posteriorly the gastrocnemius and soleus act to flex the knee and plantarflex the ankle. There are also muscles that flex the toes and ankle. The tibial nerve and artery run with these muscles.
• Laterally the peroneus longus and peroneus brevis evert the ankle.
• Anterolaterally the tibialis anterior, extensor hallucis longus and extensor digitorum longus extend (aka *dorsiflex*) the ankle, big toe and lesser toes, respectively. Similar to the thigh, the muscles are encased with tough fascia and separated by septa making compartment syndrome a risk in trauma.

Ankle

The ankle is a hinge between the talus and tibia. The talus acts as a fulcrum and is stabilised by the medial malleolus of the tibia and the lateral malleolus of the fibula. This configuration is known as a mortise. Fracture of either the lateral or medial malleoli may result in disruption of the mortise.

In addition to the bones, ligaments also stabilise the ankle. Medially is the tough deltoid ligament. Laterally there are three main ligaments: the anterior talofibular ligament, the calcaneofibular ligament and the posterior talofibular ligament. Inversion injuries can tear or stretch the lateral ligament complex, resulting in an ankle sprain.

Foot

The foot is composed of the talus, calcaneum, navicular, cuboid, three cuneiforms, five metatarsals and 14 phalanges. On the sole of the foot flexor tendons flex the toes. Dorsally lie extensor tendons. Medially the tibialis posterior tendon inserts into the navicular and supports the arch as well as providing inversion. Laterally the peroneus brevis inserts into the base of the fifth metatarsal to evert the foot. Fracture of this bony insertion occurs after inversion injury and is prone to non-union.

10 Clinical anatomy of the spine

Figure 10.1   The anatomy of a lumbar vertebra

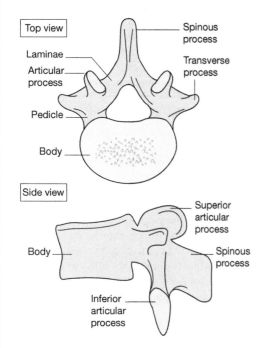

Top view

Spinous process

Laminae

Transverse process

Articular process

Pedicle

Body

Side view

Body

Superior articular process

Spinous process

Inferior articular process

Figure 10.2   Differences between vertebrae

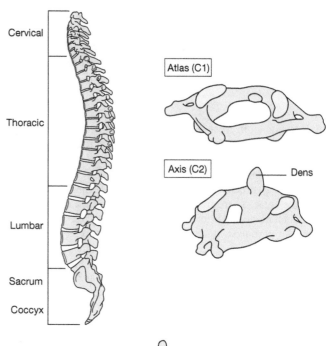

Cervical

Thoracic

Lumbar

Sacrum

Coccyx

Atlas (C1)

Axis (C2)

Dens

Cervical
Small size
Transverse foramena
Rudimentary transverse process
Flat facets

Thoracic
Larger size
Larger transverse processes articulating with ribs
Oblique facets

Lumbar
Largest size
Stout transverse processes
Almost vertical facets

Figure 10.3   Spinal ligaments

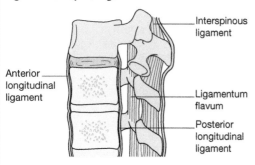

Interspinous ligament

Anterior longitudinal ligament

Ligamentum flavum

Posterior longitudinal ligament

Figure 10.4   Intervertebral discs

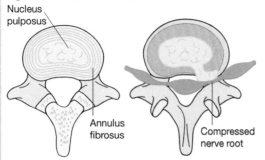

Nucleus pulposus

Annulus fibrosus

Compressed nerve root

(a) The central nucleus pulposus is usually contained by the tough outer annulus fibrosus

(b) Herniation of the nucleus may compress adjacent nerve roots

Figure 10.5   Spinal tracts The nerves are arranged in functional groups as they pass along the spinal cord

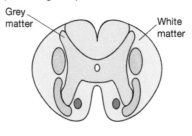

Grey matter

White matter

○ Lateral corticospinal tract: motor
● Anterior corticospinal tract: motor
○ Dorsal column: proprioception and vibration
○ Spinothalamic: pain, touch and temperature

Figure 10.6   Relationship of disc to nerve roots

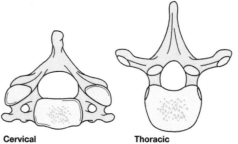
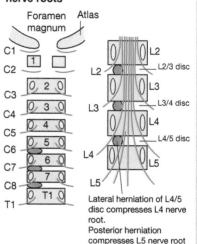

Foramen magnum   Atlas

C1
C2
C3
C4
C5
C6
C7
C8
T1

1 2 3 4 5 6 7 T1

L2
L2/3 disc
L3
L3/4 disc
L4
L4/5 disc
L5

Lateral herniation of L4/5 disc compresses L4 nerve root.
Posterior herniation compresses L5 nerve root

Trauma and Orthopaedics at a Glance, First Edition. Henry Willmott.
© 2016 John Wiley & Sons, Ltd. Published 2016 by John Wiley & Sons, Ltd. Companion website: www.ataglanceseries.com/TandO

Overview

The vertebral column provides structural support to the body and transmits body weight to the pelvis. The spinal canal is a bony cavity that contains the spinal cord, the spinal nerve roots and the meninges. The spine is divided into four segments: cervical, thoracic, lumbar and sacral. There are seven cervical vertebrae, twelve thoracic vertebrae, five lumbar vertebrae and five sacral vertebrae – the latter are fused to form a solid mass. The vertebrae within each segment have different characteristics, which allow varying amounts of flexion or rotation, and confer either lordosis or kyphosis.

Vertebrae

The size and shape of vertebrae vary between segments, but all vertebrae have common features. Anteriorly is the vertebral body. Posteriorly, the vertebral arch encloses the spinal canal in which lies the spinal cord. The vertebral arch consists of two pedicles, which arise from the vertebral body, and two flattened laminae, which come together to form the posterior wall of the arch.

The vertebral arch gives off a spinous process posteriorly, two transverse processes laterally and four articular processes, two superior and two inferior. The articular processes articulate with the corresponding processes of the vertebra above and below to form the facet joints.

The first and second cervical vertebrae (C1 and C2) are different, in that they allow a large amount of rotation of the head. Their structure is therefore different from other vertebrae. This is discussed further in Chapter 46.

Intervertebral discs

Between adjacent vertebral bodies lie intervertebral discs. Discs allow movement between vertebral bodies and act as shock absorbers. They are composed of a tough fibrocartilaginous annulus fibrosus, surrounding a squashy nucleus pulposus made of water and cartilage. As an individual gets older the fibres of the annulus fibrosus degenerate and weaken. Excessive loading of the disc may result in rupture of the annulus fibrosus and herniation of the nucleus pulposus. This may press on nerve roots or the spinal cord.

Spinal ligaments

Three main groups of ligaments connect the vertebrae to each other:
• The anterior longitudinal ligament runs as a continuous band along the anterior aspect of the vertebral bodies from skull to sacrum. It is wide and strong.
• The posterior longitudinal ligament is a band connecting the posterior aspect of the vertebral bodies. It is not as strong as the anterior longitudinal ligament but is very important as it forms the anterior boundary of the spinal canal. If the posterior longitudinal ligament is disrupted in the event of a vertebral body fracture, bone fragments may encroach into the canal, possibly resulting in cord compression.
• The third important group of ligaments are the interspinous ligaments, which run between adjacent spinous processes. They act like guyropes to prevent excessive forward flexion of the spine.

Spinal cord

The spinal cord runs from the midbrain to the lower border of L1 in adults. Here it tapers to form the conus medullaris. A tiny thread-like elongation called the filum terminale continues to insert into the coccyx.

The cord is composed of upper motor neurones and sensory neurones. The nerves are arranged into tracts. Each tract has a different function.

Spinal nerves

Along the course of the spinal cord are attached spinal nerve roots. Each spinal level has a corresponding pair of nerve roots. The anterior nerve roots are motor, the posterior roots sensory. The nerve roots pass laterally where they unite to form a mixed sensory and motor spinal nerve. Beyond the conus medullaris, spinal nerves continue as a leash, which resembles a horse's tail. This is called the cauda equina.

The spinal nerves exit the spinal canal through a gap between adjacent laminae, known as an intervertebral foramen. Each spinal nerve is allocated a name, based on the segment of cord from which it arises.

It is important to understand the function of each spinal nerve, in order to correlate nerve dysfunction with clinical signs.

Nerve compression

Spinal nerves can be compressed by herniated discs. It is important to appreciate which nerves can be compressed by which disc. This differs between cervical, thoracic or lumbar segments.

There are eight cervical roots but only seven cervical vertebrae. C7 nerve therefore exits between C6 and C7 vertebrae. C8 nerve exits between C7 and T1 vertebrae.

In the thoracic spine there are 12 vertebrae and 12 nerve roots. Each nerve root exits beneath the corresponding vertebra. T1 nerve therefore exits between T1 and T2.

The lumbar spine is different, in that beyond L1 the cord has terminated and the nerve roots form the cauda equina. Each nerve root traverses the posterior edge of the disc before passing through the intervertebral foramen at the level below. Therefore a herniated disc could cause nerve compression in two ways: posterior herniation compresses the traversing nerve root of the level below; lateral herniation compresses the exiting nerve root of the level above. For example, consider the L4-5 disc. If it herniates posteriorly it will compress the L5 nerve. If it herniates laterally it will compress the L4 nerve as it exits the vertebral foramen.

Examination of the upper limb

Figure 11.1   Shoulder examination

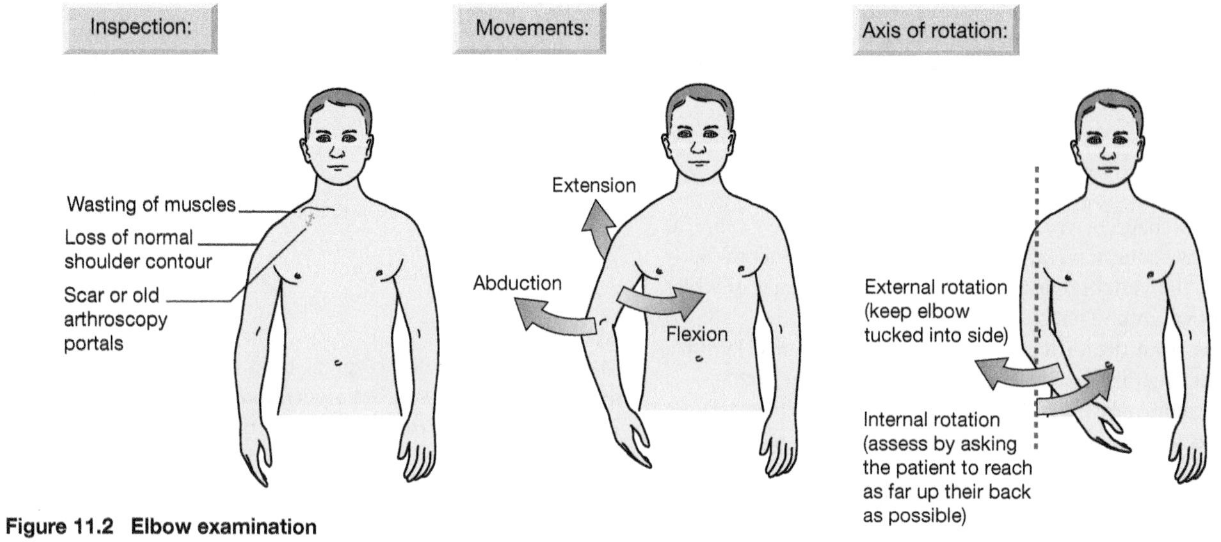

Inspection:

Wasting of muscles
Loss of normal shoulder contour
Scar or old arthroscopy portals

Movements:

Extension
Abduction
Flexion

Axis of rotation:

External rotation (keep elbow tucked into side)
Internal rotation (assess by asking the patient to reach as far up their back as possible)

Figure 11.2   Elbow examination

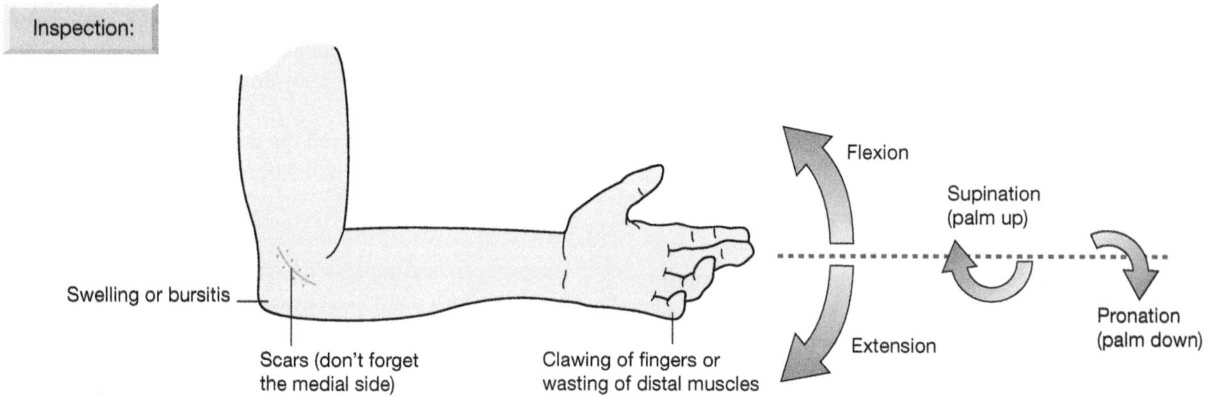

Inspection:

Swelling or bursitis
Scars (don't forget the medial side)
Clawing of fingers or wasting of distal muscles

Flexion
Extension
Supination (palm up)
Pronation (palm down)

Figure 11.3   Wrist examination

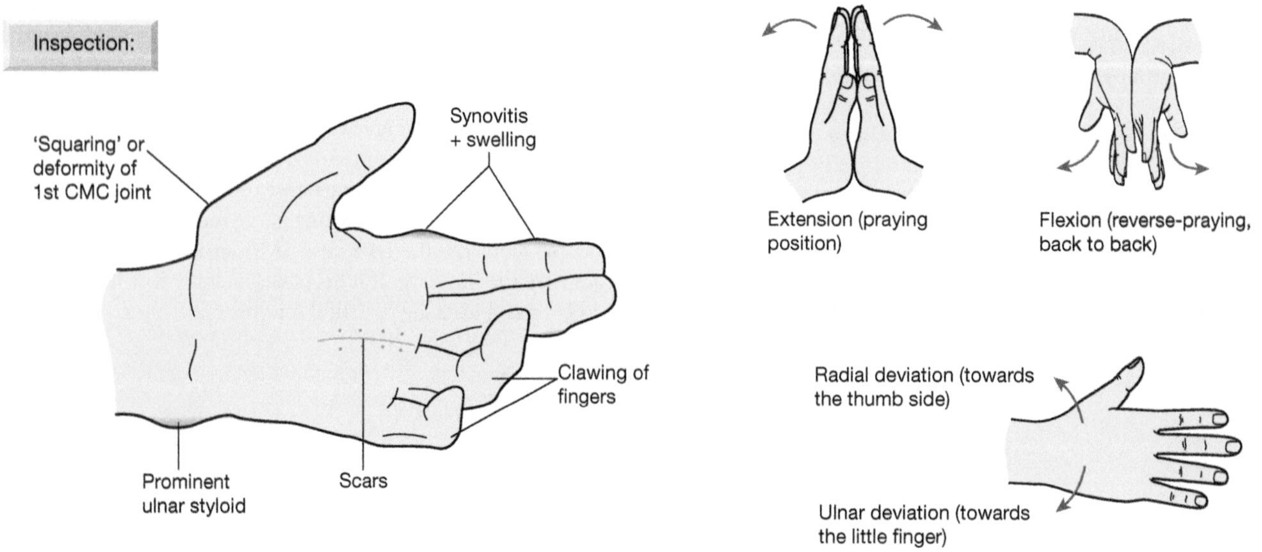

Inspection:

'Squaring' or deformity of 1st CMC joint
Synovitis + swelling
Clawing of fingers
Prominent ulnar styloid
Scars

Extension (praying position)
Flexion (reverse-praying, back to back)

Radial deviation (towards the thumb side)
Ulnar deviation (towards the little finger)

Trauma and Orthopaedics at a Glance, First Edition. Henry Willmott.
© 2016 John Wiley & Sons, Ltd. Published 2016 by John Wiley & Sons, Ltd. Companion website: www.ataglanceseries.com/TandO

General framework

Before examining a patient, take a history. Use this information, along with the patient's age, to generate a shortlist of likely diagnoses. The act of examining the patient is therefore simply to rule in or rule out those diagnoses. With practice, this will become second nature.

Prepare the patient properly for examination. Gain verbal consent. Ask for a chaperone if appropriate. Ensure the patient feels comfortable and has privacy, with curtains drawn or door closed. Expose the patient properly. For the upper limb this means removing shirts or jumpers so that both limbs can be seen together, along with the cervical and thoracic spine.

When it comes to the examination, a structured approach is essential. Stick to the framework:

- **Look**
- **Feel**
- **Move**
- **Special tests**

Shoulder

Look: Inspect for muscle **wasting**, looking especially for a hollow above the scapula where supraspinatus lies.
- Look for abnormal **posturing** of the limb and compare with the other side.
- Look for **scars**, including **arthroscopy portals**, which may be hard to see.

Feel: Sit the patient down in a chair and **stand behind them**.
- Ask them if they have **pain** and **palpate** the sternoclavicular joint, clavicle, acromioclavicular joint, the supra- and infraspinous fossae of the scapula, and across the tip of the acromion where the bursa may be inflamed. Feel for the coracoid process, and move laterally to feel the anterior aspect of the glenohumeral joint.

Move: Start with simple **screening tests**.
- Ask the patient to put their **hands on their head**. Any pathology may become obvious.
- In order to assess each movement individually stand in front of the patient and ask them to mimic your actions:
  - **forward flexion** (arm forwards);
  - **abduction** (arm out sideways);
  - **external rotation** (elbow flexed and tucked in to the side, both arms rotate outwards together for comparison);
  - **internal rotation** (measured by how far up the spine the patient can reach).

Special tests:
- For the **rotator cuff**, test:
  - **resisted abduction** (supraspinatus);
  - **resisted external rotation** (infraspinatus);
  - **resisted internal rotation** (best achieved by asking the patient to put their hand on their abdomen and press inwards, for subscapularis).
- For **instability**, test:
  - **apprehension**, by lying the patient down and bringing the arm up and out to the side. If the shoulder is unstable anteriorly, the patient will resist this movement.
- For **subacromial impingement**:
  - **Hawkin's test** puts the shoulder in flexion and adduction with the elbow flexed. Twist the shoulder in internal rotation to reproduce pain.
- Always finish the shoulder examination by examining movements of the **cervical spine** and assessing the function of the **main nerves**: radial, ulnar, median, axillary and musculocutaneous.

Elbow

Look: Look for **scars**, especially hard to see on the medial side. Check for **wasting** or **contracture** of the hand, which may represent nerve injury. Swelling and deformity of other joints may indicate rheumatoid arthritis.

Feel: **Palpate** the medial and lateral epicondyles, the olecranon and triceps tendon. Palpate the radial head (find the location on your own elbow by pronating and supinating your forearm).

Move: **Flexion, extension, pronation, supination**. The latter two should be done with the elbow held into the patient's side to prevent 'cheating' by twisting the shoulder. Compare with the other side.

Special tests: Assess **nerve** function, especially ulnar nerve, which may be compressed at the elbow. **Resisted wrist extension** may be painful in tennis elbow.

Wrist

Look: Look for **scars**, **deformity** consistent with trauma or swelling caused by rheumatoid arthritis (RA) or a ganglion. **Wasting** of the thenar muscles occurs in carpal tunnel syndrome. **Clawing** occurs with ulnar nerve injury.

Feel: **Palpate** radial styloid, the joint line, the ulnar styloid, the distal radioulnar joint (which may be unstable in RA). Palpate the tendons, feeling for warmth or tenderness suggestive of inflammation. Check the anatomical snuff box for tenderness if scaphoid injury is suspected.

Move: **Flexion and extension** may be assessed by asking the patient to put their hands in the praying position, and reverse praying position.
- **Radial and ulnar deviation** are compared with the other side.
- **Pronation and supination** may be painful if the distal radioulnar joint is unstable.

Special tests: Check the function of **median, ulnar and radial nerves.**
- Ballottement of the distal radio-ulnar joint (**DRUJ**) indicates instability.
- de Quervain's tenosynovitis of the tendons at the radial styloid results in pain exacerbated by **Finkelstein's test** (tuck the thumb into a clenched fist and ulnar deviate the wrist).

Hand

Look: Look from distal to proximal, assessing **wasting, deformity, scars** or **skin changes**. Compare with the other hand. Look for the classic **boutonnières** or **swan-neck** deformities of the fingers.

Feel: The small joints of the hand are affected in RA and they may be **warm and tender**.

Move: **Screening tests** include making a fist, making a pinch grip and holding a pencil. Assess **movement at each joint** in each finger. If a joint is contracted, check if it can be passively extended.

Special tests: Assess the deep and superficial flexor tendons of each finger.
- **Flexor digitorum profundus (FDP)** is assessed by flexing the distal interphalangeal joint.
- **Flexor digitorum superficialis (FDS)** is assessed by flexing the finger at the proximal interphalangeal joint whilst holding the other fingers straight.
- **Extensors** are assessed by resisted extension.
- Each finger has a pair of **digital nerves** that should be individually checked.

Finally check the **radial and ulnar arteries** by performing an Allen's test.

12 Examination of the lower limb

Figure 12.1 Assessment of the gait cycle
Ensure adequate exposure and walk the patient to and fro.
Assess for use of orthoses, pain and relative length of stance and swing phase

	Stance (60%)				Swing (40%)		
Initial contact	Loading response	Mid-stance	Terminal stance	Pre-swing	Initial swing	Mid-swing	Terminal swing

Figure 12.2 Hip examination
(a) Trendelenberg test. Stand on the affected limb, support the patient with your hands, feel for weight shift, watch for pelvic tilt
(b) Thomas' test. Obliterate the lumbar lordosis by flexing the unaffected limb. Assess for full extension
(c) Assess extent of flexion, and internal and external rotation

(a)
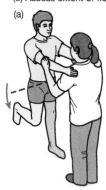

(b)
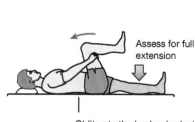

Assess for full extension

Obliterate the lumbar lordosis by flexing the unaffected limb

(c)
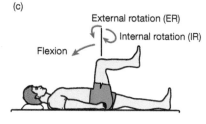

External rotation (ER)
Internal rotation (IR)
Flexion

Figure 12.3 Knee examination
(a) Inspect from behind looking for scars and alignment.
Varus is bow-legs, valgus is knock-knees

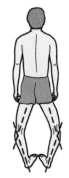

(b) On the couch assess flexion and extension
Special tests include posterior sag (PCL) and anterior drawer (ACL)

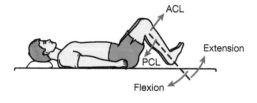

ACL
Extension
PCL
Flexion

Figure 12.4 Foot and ankle examination
(a) Inspect from behind.
Assess spine for signs of spina bifida
Check hind foot alignment.
Stand patient on tiptoes to assess tibialis posterior function

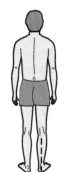

(b) Assess movements
Ankle flexion and extension, subtalar inversion and eversion and mid-foot pronation and supination

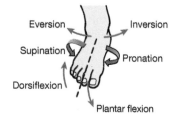

Eversion
Inversion
Supination
Pronation
Dorsiflexion
Plantar flexion

Trauma and Orthopaedics at a Glance, First Edition. Henry Willmott.
© 2016 John Wiley & Sons, Ltd. Published 2016 by John Wiley & Sons, Ltd. Companion website: www.ataglanceseries.com/TandO

Gait

All examinations of the lower limbs should start by **asking the patient to walk**.

Assess the gait pattern with the patient **properly exposed** so that the **inclination of the pelvis** can be seen clearly. Walk them towards and away. Note the use of any **aids** such as a stick.

Break the gait cycle down into a separate stance phase and swing phase.

An **antalgic** gait is a shortened stance phase due to pain. A **leg length discrepancy** causes the patient to vault over the short limb. Spasticity after a stroke may result in a **circumduction gait**. A foot drop causes a **high-stepping gait** and the affected foot will slap onto the floor. Abductor weakness gives a waddling **Trendelenburg gait**.

Hip

Look: With the patient standing, look for **wasting** of the abductors (gluteii). **Scars** may be well healed. Old **sinuses** represent infection. Look around the knee or heel for scars left by skeletal traction pins, which was how femoral and pelvic fractures were treated historically.

Special tests: in a break to the look, feel, move, special test framework, when examining the hip it is easier to do a **Trendelenburg test** before the patient lies on the couch. This tests abductor power.
- Stand facing the patient.
- Offer them your hands for support.
- Ask them to stand on the good leg, then the bad.
- **Watch for the pelvis tilting downwards** on the opposite side to the weak muscles ('the sound side sags'). In subtle cases, the pelvic tilt may not be obvious, but the increased pressure exerted by the patient on your hands is easily felt.

Thomas' test is another 'special test' that must come before movements are assessed. It is used to exclude fixed flexion.
- **Lie the patient down.**
- Ask them to **pull the unaffected leg up to their chest**, using their hands to help if they wish.
- Feel under the lumbar spine to ensure any **lordosis** has been obliterated.
- Ask them to **push the knee of the affected leg into the couch.** This will reveal any fixed flexion.

Move: Following on directly from Thomas' test:
- Assess **flexion of the hip**.
- In 90° flexion assess **internal and external rotation**, remembering that this may be painful in arthritis.
- Assess **abduction** in extension.
  Measure leg lengths:
- Distance from the anterior superior iliac spine (ASIS) to the medial malleolus is the true leg length. Distance from a midline structure, such as the umbilicus is apparent leg length, caused by abduction contracture.
- Apparent leg length discrepancy is rarely seen and of doubtful clinical relevance, but it seems to come up in exams!

Finally check the **neurovascular status of the legs and assess the spine**.

Knee

Look: With the patient **standing** assess for:
- **Varus** (bow-leg).
- **Valgus** (knock-knee) deformity.
- This is done most easily from behind.
- Also look for **scars and swelling**, including behind the knee (Baker's cyst). **Quadriceps wasting** is common.

Feel: Check for an **effusion** using the patella tap test or the medial bulge test.

- **Palpate for tenderness:** Bend the knee to around 60° and stabilise it by sitting on the couch to prevent the patient's foot from moving. Palpate systematically starting at the tibial tuberosity, patellar tendon, prepatellar bursa, quadriceps tendon, medial joint line, medial collateral ligament, lateral joint line and lateral collateral ligament.

Move: Check range of **flexion and extension**, assessing for a fixed flexion deformity. As you move the knee **feel for crepitus**.

Special tests: Assess the integrity of the collateral ligaments by exerting a **varus and valgus stress**. This is best done by holding the tibia securely under your arm against your own flank. By moving your own pelvis you can easily exert varus/valgus force.

Assess the **anterior (ACL) and posterior (PCL) cruciate ligaments:**
- **PCL:** The posterior cruciate prevents posterior subluxation of the tibia. With both knees bent to 90° push the tibia backwards and see how far the tibia sags backwards compared to the other side.
- **ACL:** In the same position, pull the tibia forwards to perform the **anterior draw test**. Excessive anterior movement indicates that the ACL may be damaged. A more sensitive test is **Lachmann's test**. This involves gripping the femur with one hand and the tibia with the other. In 30° flexion, try and elicit anterior and posterior subluxation and feel for the end point. This test is difficult, especially in large patients.

The final special test is **McMurray's test for meniscal tears**. It is a painful test and not particularly sensitive. It involves flexing the knee, applying axial compression and rotation whilst extending the knee, feeling for a painful click.

Ankle

Look: Always inspect the foot and ankle with the **patient standing**.
- Look for **swelling** around the ankle or in the joints of the foot.
- Assess the **arches**, noting whether the foot is flat or has a very high arch.
- Assess **heel alignment**: normally the heel is in slight valgus.
- Whilst looking from behind ask the patient to **stand on tiptoes** whilst standing only on one foot. Normally this should bring the heel into varus. This assesses tibialis posterior.
- **Look at the sole**, assessing for **callosities or ulcers**.
- Inspect the **toes** looking for **bunions** (hallux valgus), **clawing or hammering** of the toes.
- Whilst the patient is standing, look at the **base of the spine**, checking for a dimple or naevus, which may represent **spina bifida**.

Feel: Palpate systematically, starting behind the medial malleolus to assess tibialis posterior inflammation. Move to the medial joint line where swelling and inflammation from the ankle joint may be evident. Move across the anterior joint, down to the tip of the fibula and back to the peroneal tendons. Feel the base of the fifth metatarsal for pain associated with a fracture here. Finally examine the midfoot and toes, assessing for synovitis.

Move: Assess three joints separately:
- **Tibiotalar** (ankle): ankle movements are flexion and extension, often referred to as dorsiflexion and plantarflexion.
- **Subtalar:** subtalar movements are varus and valgus. Assess these by gripping the calcaneum with one hand and the ankle with the other.
- **Midfoot:** the midfoot allows pronation and supination, assessed by holding the calcaneum still and moving the forefoot.

Assess the **power** of tibialis anterior (ankle extension), **tibialis posterior** (foot inversion), **peroneii** (foot eversion) and **gastrocnemius/soleus** (ankle flexion).

Special tests: Ankle instability may lead to laxity of the ankle, which can be assessed by performing an **anterior draw test**. Stabilise the tibia and pull the foot forwards, comparing with the other side.
- Check dorsalis pedis and posterior tibial **pulses**.
- Assess for presence of **peripheral neuropathy**, especially in diabetic patients.

13 Examination of the spine

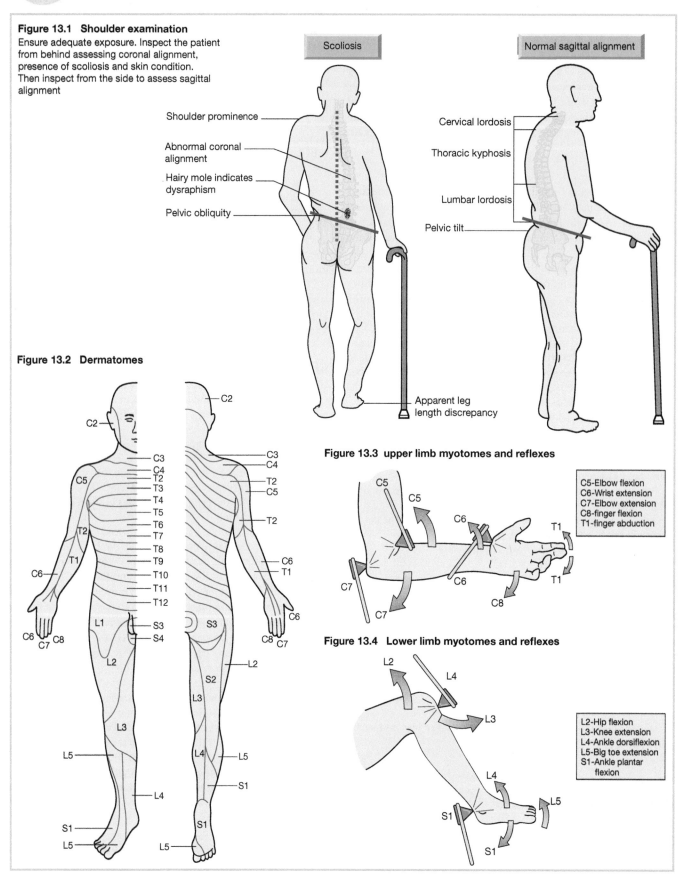

Figure 13.1 Shoulder examination
Ensure adequate exposure. Inspect the patient from behind assessing coronal alignment, presence of scoliosis and skin condition. Then inspect from the side to assess sagittal alignment

Scoliosis

Normal sagittal alignment

Shoulder prominence

Abnormal coronal alignment

Hairy mole indicates dysraphism

Pelvic obliquity

Cervical lordosis

Thoracic kyphosis

Lumbar lordosis

Pelvic tilt

Apparent leg length discrepancy

Figure 13.2 Dermatomes

Figure 13.3 upper limb myotomes and reflexes

C5-Elbow flexion
C6-Wrist extension
C7-Elbow extension
C8-finger flexion
T1-finger abduction

Figure 13.4 Lower limb myotomes and reflexes

L2-Hip flexion
L3-Knee extension
L4-Ankle dorsiflexion
L5-Big toe extension
S1-Ankle plantar flexion

Trauma and Orthopaedics at a Glance, First Edition. Henry Willmott.
© 2016 John Wiley & Sons, Ltd. Published 2016 by John Wiley & Sons, Ltd. Companion website: www.ataglanceseries.com/TandO

Spine examination

Follow the 'look, feel, move' framework.

Look: Fully expose the patient, asking them to stand in their underwear. Look carefully from behind for pelvic tilt, scoliosis, symmetry of the shoulders and wasting of muscles. From the side inspect for the normal alignment of the spine.

The cervical spine has a natural lordosis, the thoracic spine kyphosis and the lumbar spine lordosis. The spine should be balanced in both planes. An imaginary plumb line from the C7 spinous process should pass through the top of the natal cleft.

Feel: Palpate the midline, feeling for steps and assessing for tenderness. Feel the paraspinal muscles for tenderness or spasm. Palpate the sacroiliac joints.

Move: Active movements may be assessed separately in the cervical, thoracic and lumbar segments.

It should be noted that in the context of trauma, movements should not be performed until bony injury has been excluded. See Chapter 37 for an overview of this.

In the cervical spine assess:
- Flexion and extension, by asking the patient to touch their chin on their chest and look to the ceiling.
- Rotation, by asking the patient to look to the left and right.
- Lateral flexion, by asking the patient to touch each ear to the shoulder.

In the thoracic spine assess rotation: stabilise the pelvis by asking the patient to sit on the edge of the couch and twist to either side. Folding the arms makes assessment of rotation more accurate.

In the lumbar spine assess:
- Lateral flexion: sliding the hands down the outside of each leg, recording how far the patient can reach.
- Flexion and extension: ask the patient to bend to touch their toes and then lean backwards. Movements can be accurately assessed by placing your fingers on the spinous processes of the lumbar spine so as to feel the movement of the vertebrae.

Neurological examination

Examination of the upper and lower limbs should be performed with respect to the function of the spinal nerves at each level.

Power

The examination findings are recorded in numerical form using the MRC power grading:

0 – no movement
1 – flicker of movement
2 – active movement with gravity eliminated
3 – active movement against gravity
4 – mild weakness
5 – normal
NT – not testable due to concomitant injury or immobilisation.

Upper limb
Myotomes
C5 – elbow flexion
C6 – wrist extension
C7 – elbow extension
C8 – finger flexion
T1 – finger abduction.
Reflexes
C5 – biceps tendon
C6 – supinator tendon at the wrist
C7 – triceps tendon.
Sensation
Assess light touch and pinprick in each dermatome (see Figure 13.3). This is a very subjective measure and patients sometimes find it difficult to determine what is 'normal'. Before each dermatome is tested, use the same stimulus to touch the top of the sternum, providing the patient with a benchmark.

Lower limbs
Myotomes
Power is measured in the same way as in the upper limbs The myotomes are:
L2 – hip flexion
L3 – knee extension
L4 – ankle dorsiflexion
L5 – big toe extension
S1 – ankle plantar flexion.
Reflexes
L4 – patellar tendon
S1 – Achilles tendon.
Sensation
Measured in the same way following the dermatome map (see Figure 13.4).

Rectal examination and perianal sensation

The sacral nerve roots below S1 are assessed by measuring power in the levator ani muscle, which is innervated by S2, 3 and 4. Sensation around the anus is supplied by S3, 4 and 5 in concentric rings. Remember that each sacral root is a pair, left and right. Check sensation on both the right and left sides of the midline.

Root tension signs

In patients with back pain, it may be unclear whether pain in the back of the legs is simple referred mechanical pain from the spine itself or caused by impingement of a lumbar nerve due to a disc prolapse causing sciatica. A provocative test is the straight leg raise.

- With the patient lying flat, slowly **lift the affected leg straight up off the bed**. This stretches the sciatic nerve and may provoke a shooting pain in the leg. The **angle** at which sciatica is provoked should be noted. **Allow the leg to drop by 10°** and maintaining this angle, **bring the foot into maximal dorsiflexion**. If this provokes the pain again, this is known as a root tension sign.

- A similar test exists for the femoral nerve in which the patient is **prone and the hip brought into extension**. This is rarely performed in practice.

14 The brachial plexus

Figure 14.1 Anatomy of the brachial plexus

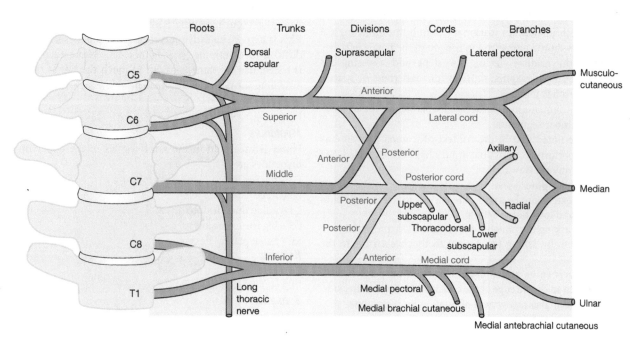

Roots | Trunks | Divisions | Cords | Branches

Dorsal scapular
Suprascapular
Lateral pectoral
C5
Anterior
Musculo-cutaneous
C6
Superior
Lateral cord
Anterior
Posterior
Axillary
C7
Middle
Posterior cord
Posterior
Median
Posterior
Upper subscapular
Radial
Posterior
Thoracodorsal
Lower subscapular
C8
Inferior
Anterior
Medial cord
T1
Long thoracic nerve
Medial pectoral
Ulnar
Medial brachial cutaneous
Medial antebrachial cutaneous

Figure 14.2 Erb's palsy
Upper brachial plexus avulsion injury
(a) Mechanisms of injury:

1. Shoulder dystocia during delivery

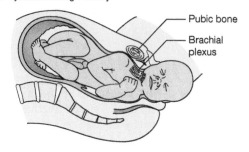

Pubic bone

Brachial plexus

2. Fall onto shoulder with extreme lateral flexion of neck

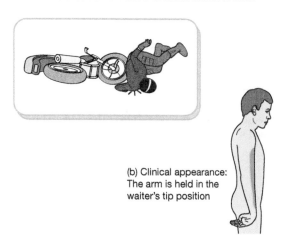

(b) Clinical appearance: The arm is held in the waiter's tip position

Figure 14.3 Klumpke's palsy
Lower brachial plexus avulsion injury

(a) Mechanism of injury: person catching themselves in a fall

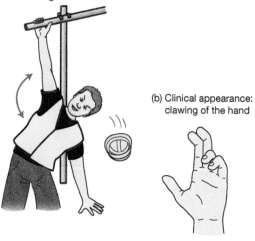

(b) Clinical appearance: clawing of the hand

(c) If the sympathetic chain is avulsed, Horner's syndrome may result

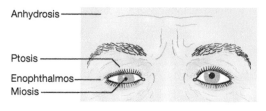

Anhydrosis

Ptosis

Enophthalmos

Miosis

Trauma and Orthopaedics at a Glance, First Edition. Henry Willmott.
© 2016 John Wiley & Sons, Ltd. Published 2016 by John Wiley & Sons, Ltd. Companion website: www.ataglanceseries.com/TandO

Anatomy

The brachial plexus is a network of interconnecting nerves at the root of the neck. Although at first the structure is complex, knowledge of the layout is helpful in understanding the sequelae of brachial plexus injury.

It is formed from the C5–T1 nerve roots and is divided into five sections:
- Roots
- Trunks
- Divisions
- Cords
- Branches

The mnemonic 'Remember To Drink Cold Beer' will help.

The brachial plexus has five roots from C5 to T1.

There are three trunks, named superior, middle and inferior. The superior and inferior trunks each have two contributing roots, the middle trunk has only one.

Each trunk then divides into anterior and posterior divisions.

The cords are named with respect to their relationship to the brachial artery in the axilla. All the posterior divisions combine to form the posterior cord. The lateral cord is formed from the anterior divisions of the superior and middle trunks, and the medial cord is a continuation of the anterior division of the inferior trunk.

There are five terminal branches:

- **Musculocutaneous nerve** – mixed sensory and motor, supplies muscles in the anterior compartment of the arm including biceps and brachialis before terminating as the medial cutaneous nerve of the forearm.
- **Radial nerve** – innervates extensor muscles of the arm, forearm and fingers and supplies sensation to the dorsal first webspace.
- **Axillary nerve** – supplies motor power to deltoid and teres minor and sensation to the skin overlying the deltoid (regimental badge area).
- **Ulnar nerve** – motor to the flexor carpi ulnaris, half of flexor digitorum profundus (FDP) and intrinsic muscles of the hand, sensory to the ulnar one-and-a-half digits.
- **Median nerve** – motor to most of the flexor muscles of the forearm and the LOAF muscles of the thenar eminence, sensory to the radial three-and-a-half digits.

Note: LOAF is an *aide mémoire* to remember the muscles innervated by the median nerve:

Lateral two lumbricals
Opponens pollicis
Abductor pollicis brevis
Flexor pollicis brevis

There are ten lesser branches:

- **Nerve to subclavius** – a tiny filament supplying the subclavius muscle underneath the clavicle. Of no clinical significance.
- **Dorsal scapular nerve** – motor to the rhomboids of the back.
- **Upper subscapular nerve** – innervates the superior half of subscapularis.
- **Lower subscapular nerve** – supplies the inferior half of subscapularis and teres major of the rotator cuff.
- **Long thoracic nerve** – arising from C5, 6 and 7 roots just after they emerge from the neural foramina, it supplies motor power to serratus anterior. Injury results in winging of the scapula.
- **Suprascapular nerve** – supplies infraspinatus and supraspinatus muscles of the rotator cuff.
- **Lateral pectoral nerve** – innervates the lateral head of pectoralis major.
- **Medial pectoral nerve** – innervates pectoralis minor and the medial head of pectoralis major.
- **Medial brachial cutaneous nerve** – sensory supply to the posterior and medial aspects of the arm as far as the elbow.
- **Medial antebrachial cutaneous nerve** – supplies sensation to the medial aspect of the forearm.

Injuries to the brachial plexus

The brachial plexus is well protected by the clavicle and is encased by muscle. Injuries are rare, but when they do occur, are caused by significant trauma. If the arm is forced into extreme positions, the brachial plexus may be stretched resulting in tearing of the nerve fibres or avulsion of the nerve roots from the spinal cord. There are three classic patterns of injury:

- **Erb's palsy:** Extreme lateral flexion of the neck combined with depression of the shoulder, such as a fall onto the shoulder or shoulder dystocia during delivery in an infant, results in traction of the superior part of the plexus. The C5 and C6 roots are affected, resulting in loss of axillary, suprascapular, musculocutaneous and radial nerves. The arm is held adducted, internally rotated, pronated and extended at elbow in the 'waiter's tip' position.
- **Klumpke's palsy:** Extreme abduction of the arm, such as catching oneself in a fall from a height, results in injury to the lower roots. The median and ulnar nerves are affected and the hand is clawed. If the nerve roots are avulsed from the spinal cord, the sympathetic chain may be affected, resulting in Horner's syndrome (miosis, ptosis, enophthalmos and anhidrosis). This has a poor prognosis.
- **Complete:** A rare injury caused by massive trauma; all nerve roots are injured, resulting in flaccid paralysis of the arm. The prognosis is usually very poor.

Penetrating injuries: Gunshot wounds or stabbings to the neck region may result in injury to any part of the plexus. A haematoma following brachial artery injury may put pressure on the plexus. Progressive neurological symptoms may indicate an expanding haematoma.

Management

The first priority is to establish the location of the injury. Careful neurological examination of the upper limb is essential, testing each branch individually. Chest X-ray and cervical spine X-rays are also helpful to look for a raised diaphragm indicating phrenic nerve injury and transverse process fractures of the cervical spine indicating traction injury. MRI will demonstrate gross injury to the plexus or avulsion of nerve roots from the cervical spinal cord.

Most cases are observed for at least 6 weeks to allow for any spontaneous recovery. Indications for immediate exploration of the plexus are penetrating injuries (except gunshot wounds, which are usually managed conservatively), iatrogenic injuries, open injuries or progressive neurology associated with an expanding haematoma.

Delayed surgery is conducted at specialist centres and may involve a combination of direct nerve repair, nerve transfer directly to muscles, or tendon transfers whereby functioning muscles are used to take over the tasks of muscles that are not working.

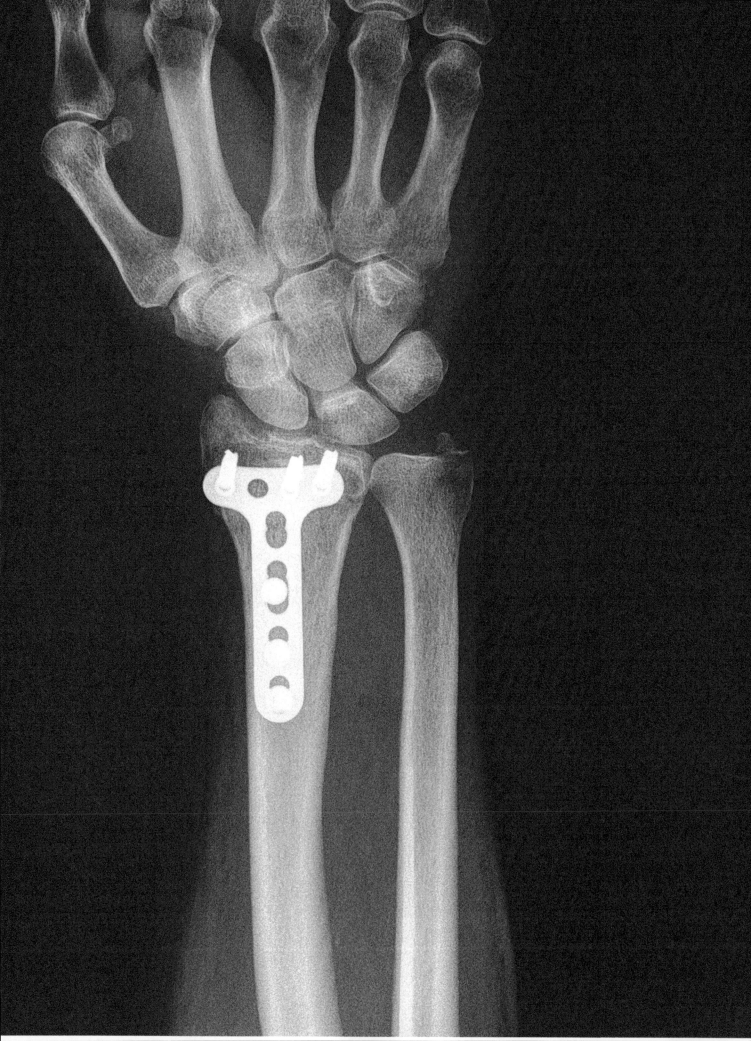

Adult orthopaedics

Part 2

Chapters

 Visit the companion website at www.ataglanceseries.com/TandO to test yourself on these topics.

Shoulder 1

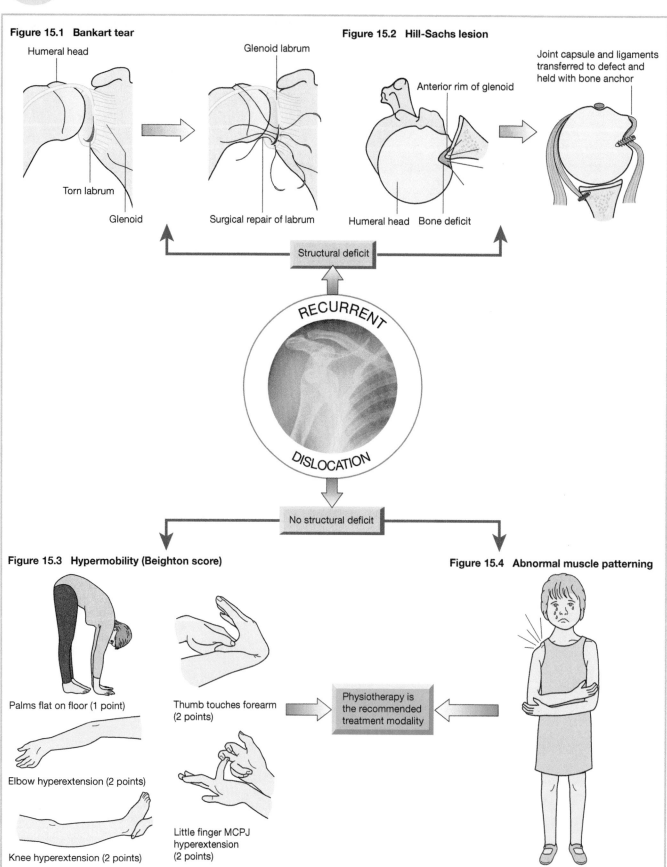

Figure 15.1 Bankart tear

Humeral head

Glenoid labrum

Torn labrum

Glenoid

Surgical repair of labrum

Figure 15.2 Hill-Sachs lesion

Anterior rim of glenoid

Joint capsule and ligaments transferred to defect and held with bone anchor

Humeral head   Bone deficit

Structural deficit

RECURRENT

DISLOCATION

No structural deficit

Figure 15.3 Hypermobility (Beighton score)

Palms flat on floor (1 point)

Thumb touches forearm (2 points)

Elbow hyperextension (2 points)

Knee hyperextension (2 points)

Little finger MCPJ hyperextension (2 points)

Physiotherapy is the recommended treatment modality

Figure 15.4 Abnormal muscle patterning

Trauma and Orthopaedics at a Glance, First Edition. Henry Willmott.
© 2016 John Wiley & Sons, Ltd. Published 2016 by John Wiley & Sons, Ltd. Companion website: www.ataglanceseries.com/TandO

Problems related to instability

Acute dislocations are covered in Chapter 38. Sequelae following a dislocation can occur, and shoulder instability in itself can be problematic, even in the absence of a frank dislocation.

Rotator cuff tear

The rotator cuff muscles are a group of four muscles that form a hood around the proximal humerus. They comprise:

- **supraspinatus – abducts in the plane of the scapula (30°);**
- **subscapularis – internally rotates humerus;**
- **infraspinatus – externally rotates humerus;**
- **teres minor – externally rotates humerus in abduction.**

It is important to differentiate between an acute and a chronic cuff tear.

A chronic cuff tear may occur in the elderly without any history of trauma, due to degeneration of the tendons. Chronic cuff tears are discussed separately in Chapter 16.

Acute cuff tears are the result of an injury to a previously normal cuff. They are common after dislocation in middle-aged patients. The patient complains of pain and weakness.

Examination will reveal weakness in one or more elements of the rotator cuff. Abduction, external rotation and internal rotation should each be tested in turn. X-rays should be performed to exclude a fracture, followed by either ultrasound or MRI to delineate the tendons of the rotator cuff.

Results of repair are better if performed within 3 months of the injury. Repair can be performed either by open surgery or arthroscopic means. There is some evidence that patients return to work more quickly following arthroscopic repair, although function is equal after 6 months.

Structural defects resulting in repeat dislocation

When a shoulder is dislocated, the glenoid or the head of the humerus can be damaged. Sometimes this results in an unstable shoulder that frequently dislocates, even with very minimal force.

The cartilaginous labrum, which runs around the rim of the glenoid and serves to deepen it, can be torn off. This is known as a **Bankart lesion**. If it is associated with a 'chip' off the rim of the glenoid it is called a **bony-Bankart lesion**. Both can be associated with recurrent dislocations and, if this is the case, should be repaired.

Investigations include a CT to evaluate bone loss, or an MRI arthrogram, in which contrast is injected into the shoulder joint before an MRI is performed. The contrast can be seen leaking out of the shoulder through the tear in the labrum.

Bankart and small bony-Bankart lesions can be repaired arthroscopically. If there is a very large bony-Bankart, it may be more appropriate to perform an open operation. There are a number of operations to address a large bony defect of the glenoid. One such option is a Bristow–Latarjet procedure. In this operation the tip of the coracoid process, along with the conjoint tendon, is removed and screwed onto the front of the glenoid. This extra piece of bone 'builds up' the front of the glenoid, and helps prevent future anterior dislocations.

Sometimes the head of the humerus can be damaged after a dislocation. The humeral head is relatively soft bone and if it is dislocated anteriorly, the relatively hard glenoid can dig out a 'divot' in the humeral head. This is called a **Hill–Sachs lesion**. The resulting bone defect can sometimes be quite large. As the shoulder is brought into external rotation, the glenoid 'falls into' the defect, resulting in recurrent dislocations that are difficult to reduce. This is known as an 'engaging Hill–Sachs lesion'.

The treatment is an open surgical procedure to transfer the joint capsule and ligaments into the defect. They are held with a bone anchor. The result is to fill the defect and limit external rotation, which in itself makes dislocation less likely.

Hypermobility

Hypermobility is a common cause of shoulder problems in younger patients. The commonest form is generalised hypermobility syndrome. It is commonest in adolescent girls, and may be due to the effects of sex hormones on soft tissues. Patients tend to grow out of this and it is rarely a problem in adults. There are a number of hypermobility syndromes, such as Marfan's or Ehlers–Danlos syndrome, in which abnormal collagen causes lifelong hypermobility.

The diagnosis of hypermobility is made using the **Beighton scoring system**:

---

1 point for each side, left or right:
- Hyperextension of little finger MCPJ beyond 90°
- Hyperextension of elbow beyond 10°
- Thumb can be dorsiflexed to flexor surface of forearm
- Knee hyperextension beyond 10°

Plus one point for:
- Palms touch flat on floor with knees straight

Total out of 9. Score >4 is abnormal.

Hypermobility may result in recurrent dislocations and pain due to excessive movement beyond the physiological range.

The treatment of hypermobility syndrome and its related shoulder problems is physiotherapy. Structural defects may coexist, especially after recurrent dislocations, and these may require surgical treatment. Physiotherapy aims to strengthen the stabilising muscle groups and increase proprioception. This is the unconscious awareness of the joint's position in space so that the muscle stabilisers are activated to maintain stability.

Abnormal muscle patterning

There is a small group of patients who lose the normal coordinated action of the muscles around the shoulder so that despite the shoulder being structurally normal, it dislocates recurrently. A small cohort of patients may learn how to do this 'on demand' for psychological reasons. Once structural defects have been ruled out, the treatment is specialist physiotherapy and sometimes psychiatric involvement. It is important that the patient and their family realise that the solution to the problem lies with the patient themselves and that with support, the problem can be solved.

16 Shoulder 2

Figure 16.1 Subacromial impingement
(a) The subacromial space is between the greater tuberosity and the tip of the inferior edge of the acromion and is occupied by the suprasinatus tendon and subacromial bursa

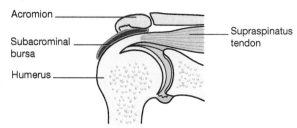

(b) A combination of an overhanging acromial tip, an enlarged or arthritic acomioclavicular joint, a thickened tendon and an inflamed bursa results in impingement when the arm is abducted. Internal rotation of the arm exacerbates the problem by forcing the greater tuberosity into the space.

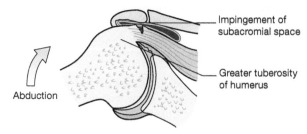

(c) Hawkins test: Abduction, flexion and internal rotation of the arm results in pain at the tip of the acromion

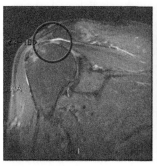

(d) Treatment includes steroid injections to reduce swelling or surgical resection of the inferior and anterior acromion.

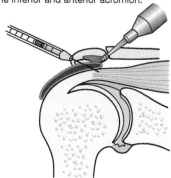

Figure 16.2 MRI scan of cuff tear
T1-weighted coronal view of the shoulder showing a tear in the supraspinatus tendon

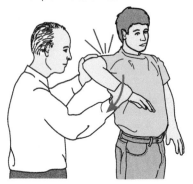

Figure 16.4 Frozen shoulder
(a) Normal shoulder: The capsule is lax and allows movement.

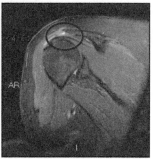

Figure 16.3
(a) Osteoarthritis of the shoulder. Note loss of joint space, subchondral sclerosis and osteophytes. The patient had pain and restricted external rotation and abduction. (b) Shoulder replacement.

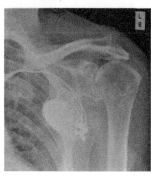
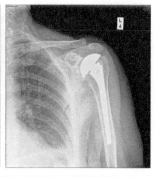

(b) Frozen shoulder: Fibrosis and contraction of the shoulder capsule results in pain and global restriction of movements. X-rays are normal

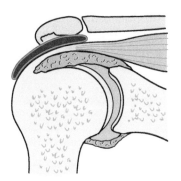

Trauma and Orthopaedics at a Glance, First Edition. Henry Willmott.
© 2016 John Wiley & Sons, Ltd. Published 2016 by John Wiley & Sons, Ltd. Companion website: www.ataglanceseries.com/TandO

Subacromial impingement

The tendon of supraspinatus runs through a narrow space between the head of the humerus and the underside of the acromion and acromioclavicular joint. It may become pinched within this space, causing pain, especially when the patient tries to perform overhead activities. This is known as subacromial impingement.

There are a number of reasons why impingement may occur. The tendon itself may become thickened either as a result of degeneration, partial tears or inflammation. The subacromial space may become narrowed due to bone spurs resulting from arthritis of the acromioclavicular joint. Some people have a naturally down-sloping acromion, which predisposes them to impingement.

The patient complains of pain, worse with repetitive overhead work. Plasterers and decorators are commonly affected. As the condition progresses, night pain becomes a feature and eventually patients may be unable to raise their arm at all.

Several clinical tests exist to detect impingement. Commonly used is **Hawkins' test**, whereby the arm is held in flexion and then internally rotated. This forces the greater tuberosity up into the subacromial space, narrowing the space even further to reproduce the patient's symptoms.

Treatment involves physiotherapy, activity modification and steroid injections into the subacromial space to reduce inflammation and pain. If these measures fail, the subacromial space can be decompressed arthroscopically. Bone and inflammatory tissue is shaved from beneath the acromion to allow the tendon to move freely.

Chronic rotator cuff tear

A chronic cuff tear, in contrast to an acute cuff tear, occurs in older patients due to degeneration of the substance of the rotator cuff tendons. The exact mechanism is unclear, but several theories exist, including failure of the blood supply to the central part of the tendons, biochemical changes in collagen or long-term mechanical impingement from the acromion. The result is pain and weakness of the shoulder, exacerbated by overhead activity. It can sometimes be difficult to differentiate clinically from subacromial impingement. An ultrasound or MRI scan is helpful.

With time, the two ends of the torn tendon may retract. Long-term disuse of the muscles of the rotator cuff results in wasting and fatty degeneration. Severely retracted tears may by irreparable, resulting in chronic pain and weakness.

Cuff arthropathy

In addition to pain and weakness, chronic failure of the rotator cuff may result in a condition called cuff arthropathy.

The cuff is important not only for movements of the shoulder, but also as a stabiliser of the humeral head. Under normal conditions, the cuff holds the humeral head down snugly against the glenoid, counteracting the powerful upwards pull of the deltoid muscle. Failure of the cuff can allow the humeral head to drift superiorly away from its normal position. In addition, synovial fluid that lubricates the joint, escapes through the tear in the joint capsule. The abnormal mechanics of this situation result in destruction of the joint surfaces and progressive arthritis.

Patients complain of pain, stiffness and weakness. Plain X-rays demonstrate superior migration of the humeral head and destruction of the joint surfaces.

Treatment is difficult, because the superior migration of the humeral head precludes the use of a normal shoulder replacement. A reverse polarity shoulder replacement attempts to restore the normal centre of rotation of the joint. Results are variable.

Arthritis
Osteoarthritis

As with any synovial joint, the shoulder can be affected by osteoarthritis (OA). This may be idiopathic or result from a previous trauma or infection. Patients who have done a lot of overhead work in their life are more often affected. They complain of constant pain and a restriction in the range of movement. This is manifest as an inability to undo their bra, wipe their bottom or reach behind their back. External rotation is usually the first movement to be affected.

There are only a few conditions causing a block to passive external rotation of the shoulder: osteoarthritis, frozen shoulder or a posterior dislocation. An X-ray, including an axillary view, will reveal the diagnosis!

Conservative treatment of OA includes analgesia and physiotherapy. Surgical treatment comprises resurfacing the head of the humerus with a metal cap (resurfacing arthroplasty), replacing just the humeral head with a metal replacement (hemiarthroplasty) or replacing the entire joint, humeral head and glenoid (total shoulder replacement). There are pros and cons to each of these procedures, which are beyond the scope of this text.

Rheumatoid arthritis

Rheumatoid arthritis (RA) is the commonest inflammatory arthropathy affecting the shoulder, but crystal arthropathies, systemic lupus erythematosus (SLE) and psoriatic arthropathy may also occur. Once non-steroidal anti-inflammatory drugs (NSAIDs), disease-modifying anti-rheumatic drugs (DMARDs) and steroids have been exhausted, arthroplasty may be considered.

Frozen shoulder

Commoner in diabetics, this condition may occur spontaneously or following minor trauma or surgery to the shoulder. The exact pathophysiology is unclear but it is characterised by fibrosis and scarring of the joint capsule resulting in pain and restriction of both passive and active ranges of movement. It is usually self-limiting but recovery may take up to 2 years. Manipulation under anaesthetic, steroid injections and arthroscopic debridement may all be used to speed recovery.

Calcific tendonitis

Deposits of calcium can form within the supraspinatus tendon, causing sudden onset of severe shoulder pain. The cause is unknown but it is associated with degeneration of the tendon and subacromial impingement. It is commonest in women aged 40–60. The calcific deposits may be seen on X-ray. Treatment is analgesia, steroid injections, physio, and if these fail, arthroscopic debridement.

17 Elbow

Figure 17.1 Total elbow replacement

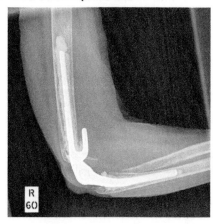

Figure 17.2 Osteoarthritis of the elbow

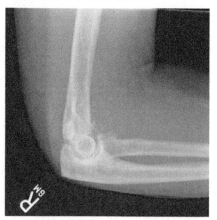

Figure 17.3 Outerbridge-Kashiwagi procedure for elbow osteoarthritis
The elbow is approached from behind and osteophytes at the posterior aspect of the elbow are debrided. A hole is then drilled through the olecranon fossa to gain access to the anterior aspect of the joint so that osteophytes at the front of the elbow are removed

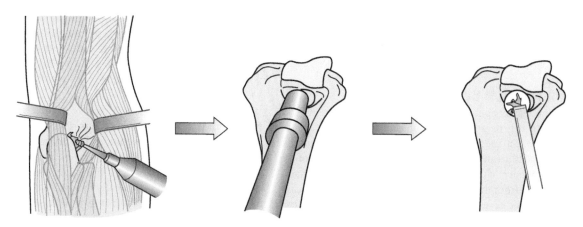

Figure 17.4 Cubital tunnel syndrome
The ulnar nerve can be trapped at five points at the elbow. The commonest point of compression is the cubital tunnel. Surgical treatment is to divide the retinacular fibres of the roof of the cubital tunnel

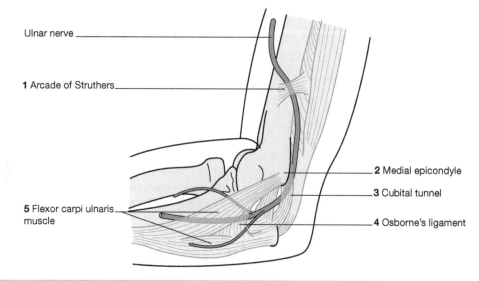

Ulnar nerve

1 Arcade of Struthers

5 Flexor carpi ulnaris muscle

2 Medial epicondyle

3 Cubital tunnel

4 Osborne's ligament

Trauma and Orthopaedics at a Glance, First Edition. Henry Willmott.
© 2016 John Wiley & Sons, Ltd. Published 2016 by John Wiley & Sons, Ltd. Companion website: www.ataglanceseries.com/TandO

Rheumatoid arthritis

Fifty percent of patients with rheumatoid arthritis (RA) have involvement of the elbow. This may manifest as:

- Painful synovitis and swelling.
- Reduction in range of movement, typically lack of full extension.
- Ulnar nerve neuropathy secondary to compression by inflamed synovium.
- Laxity of soft tissues resulting in instability.
- Destruction of articular surfaces, resulting in joint erosion, cyst formation and bone loss.

As with all joints affected by RA, the first line of treatment is to control the disease process with anti-inflammatory drugs and disease-modifying anti-rheumatic drugs (DMARDs). This is supplemented by intra-articular steroid injections. Custom-made splints may also be helpful.

Surgical treatment may consist of:

- **Elbow arthroscopy and debridement of inflamed synovium.**
- **Total elbow replacement (TER).**

Total elbow replacement is indicated when all medical treatment options have been exhausted. The complication rate is high and includes infection, wound breakdown, ulnar nerve injury and loosening of the prosthesis. It is only indicated in older or low demand patients because of concerns about the longevity of the implant. Active infection is an absolute contraindication.

Osteoarthritis

In contrast to RA, osteoarthritis (OA) of the elbow is relatively uncommon. It is typically seen in the dominant limb of manual labourers. Previous trauma is a risk factor.

The most striking feature of elbow OA is loss of movement, especially extension. This is due to contracture of the capsule and the presence of osteophytes, which limit the excursion of the olecranon. Pain is present at extremes of movement.

X-rays may show:

- Loss of joint space.
- Osteophytes.
- Subchondral sclerosis and cysts.
- Loose bodies – these may be hard to see but can cause a significant loss of movement. CT may demonstrate them more easily.

Treatment of elbow OA consists of rest, NSAIDs and activity modification. If this fails, surgical options are:

- **Arthroscopic debridement** – osteophytes are trimmed and loose bodies removed. Large osteophytes on the edge of the joint can be hard to get to.
- **Open debridement** – a number of procedures are described, but one way of removing osteophytes and freeing up the contracted capsule is the **Outerbridge–Kashiwagi procedure (OK procedure)**. This involves approaching the elbow from the posterior aspect, removing any posterior osteophytes and then carefully drilling a large hole in the thin bone at the bottom of the olecranon fossa. The anterior aspect of the joint can be accessed through this hole and any anterior osteophytes removed. The tight anterior capsule can also be released.

Tennis elbow

Lateral epicondylitis is the correct name for the condition commonly known as tennis elbow. Patients complain of pain directly over or just distal to the lateral epicondyle of the humerus. Symptoms are exacerbated by activities involving repetitive supination and extension of the wrist – such as a backhand shot in tennis.

The underlying pathophysiology is microtears of the common extensor origin, which is the broad aponeurosis from which all the extensor muscles of the forearm originate. Typically extensor carpi radialis brevis (ECRB) is most affected, although in severe cases all the extensor muscles may be involved.

Clinically symptoms are reproduced by direct pressure over the lateral epicondyle and resisted extension of the wrist and fingers.

X-rays will be normal, but ultrasound or MRI may reveal inflammation. The differential diagnosis includes entrapment of the radial nerve, so this should be carefully examined.

The mainstay of treatment is reassurance (the condition is usually self-limiting), physiotherapy and activity modification. Affected tennis players should ensure that they are fully warmed up before play, have professional coaching in technique and use a bigger racquet grip

Steroid injections into the point of maximal tenderness may be helpful. If these fail, surgical debridement of the common extensor origin is indicated. The aponeurosis is carefully split and necrotic or inflamed tissue removed. The aim is to stimulate a healing response.

Golfer's elbow

Similar to tennis elbow, this condition constitutes inflammation of the medial epicondyle and its associated common flexor/pronator mass. It is less common than tennis elbow.

Resisted pronation and wrist flexion exacerbate symptoms.

Treatment is similar to tennis elbow. Steroid injections should be used very cautiously due to proximity of the ulnar nerve, which could be damaged by a misplaced injection.

Cubital tunnel syndrome

The ulnar nerve originates from the medial cord of the brachial plexus and runs initially in the anterior compartment of the upper arm before piercing the intermuscular septum at the arcade of Struthers, 8 cm proximal to the medial epicondyle. It then runs around the back of the medial epicondyle beneath a retinaculum. This space is known as the cubital tunnel. Distally the nerve enters the forearm between the two heads of flexor carpi ulnaris (FCU), which it supplies.

The nerve may become trapped at any of these points, but the commonest site is within the cubital tunnel. Entrapment may occur due to:

- inflammation of the elbow synovium (RA);
- osteophytes or ganglia around the elbow joint (OA);
- injury to the medial collateral ligament of the elbow or overuse;
- pregnancy (generalised oedema);
- obesity;
- idiopathically.

Patients complain of sensory loss in the ulnar two-and-a-half digits and clawing due to intrinsic weakness. **Tinel's test** may be positive behind the medial condyle. Treatment is to establish the site of compression and decompress the nerve by dividing the retinaculum of the cubital tunnel.

18 Wrist and hand 1

Figure 18.1   A rheumatoid hand. Key points are

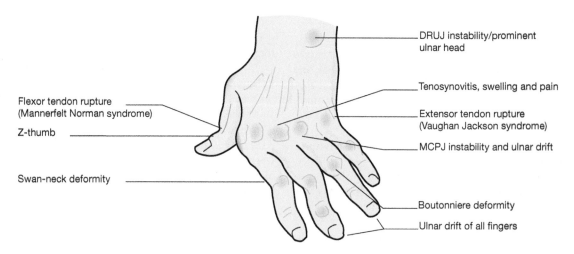

- DRUJ instability/prominent ulnar head
- Tenosynovitis, swelling and pain
- Extensor tendon rupture (Vaughan Jackson syndrome)
- MCPJ instability and ulnar drift
- Boutonniere deformity
- Ulnar drift of all fingers
- Flexor tendon rupture (Mannerfelt Norman syndrome)
- Z-thumb
- Swan-neck deformity

Figure 18.2   Boutonniere deformity

Rupture of the central slip of the extensor tendon results in flexion of the PIPJ

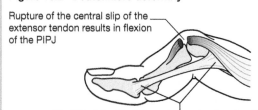

The lateral bands of the extensor tendon slip either side of the PIPJ. In this position the act flex the PIP joint and extend the DIP joint

Figure 18.3   Swan neck deformity

Rupture of the insertion of the extensor tendon into the terminal phalynx results in DIPJ flexion

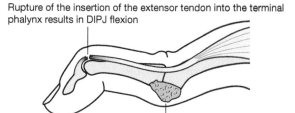

Rupture of the volar plate of the PIPJ results in hyperextension

Figure 18.4   RA hand X-ray

This AP x-ray of a hand shows several typical signs of rheumatoid arthritis. There is deformity of the thumb, with subluxation and instability at the CMC joint and the IP joint. The MCP joints of index and middle fingers are eroded and subluxed. The wrist shows extensive destruction. The bone is generally of low density and there are periarticular leucencies suggesting cyst formation

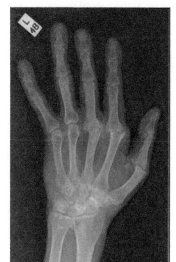

Figure 18.5   Wrist replacement x-ray

The same patient as **Figure 18.4**, with a wrist replacement in situ. The radiocarpal joint and distal radioulnar joint have both been replaced

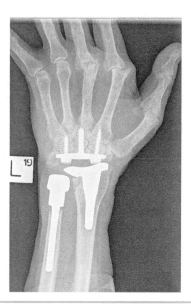

Trauma and Orthopaedics at a Glance, First Edition. Henry Willmott.
© 2016 John Wiley & Sons, Ltd. Published 2016 by John Wiley & Sons, Ltd. Companion website: www.ataglanceseries.com/TandO

Rheumatoid wrist and hand

Patients with rheumatoid arthritis (RA) commonly have involvement of the wrist and hand. There are many manifestations. The most common are:

- **Tenosynovitis** – hyperplasia of synovium surrounding the joints and tendons of the wrist and hand is common. It is a cause of swelling, warmth and pain. The inflamed tissue may exert pressure on adjacent nerves, increase the risk of tendon rupture and contribute to joint instability. Treatment consists of local steroid injections or tenosynovectomy, which is the surgical removal of inflamed synovium.
- **Extensor tendon rupture** – neglected tenosynovitis plus instability of the underlying joints can cause attrition rupture of extensor tendons. The commonest site of rupture is over the radiocarpal joint on the dorsum of the wrist. The extensor tendon to the little finger is first affected, causing drooping of the little finger (Vaughan-Jackson syndrome). Neighbouring tendons may be sequentially affected. The tendon is usually irreparable, but intact adjacent tendons can be woven into the stub of the ruptured tendon to act as a tendon-transfer.
- **Flexor tendon rupture** – less common than extensor tendon rupture, any of the flexor tendons may rupture due to inflammation and attrition. The most commonly affected is the flexor pollicis longus tendon resulting in loss of thumb flexion, known as Mannerfelt–Norman syndrome. Treatment is fusion of the thumb interphalangeal joint or tendon transfer.
- **Carpal tunnel syndrome** – hyperplastic synovium within the carpal tunnel causes compression of the median nerve, resulting in painful numbness in the thumb, index and middle finger. Treatment is carpal tunnel decompression combined with synovectomy.
- **Instability of the wrist** – chronic synovitis of the joints around the wrist eventually causes rupture of the ligaments that stabilise the carpal bones. The gap between scaphoid and lunate bones widens, the joint may sublux dorsally and in severe cases dislocate. Treatment depends on the severity of the disease but may include fusion (arthrodesis) of the wrist joint using a pin or a plate or replacement of the wrist joint (wrist arthroplasty). Patients have better range of movement with arthroplasty but a lower complication rate with arthrodesis.
- **Ulnar head subluxation** (caput ulnae syndrome) – attenuation of the ligaments that stabilise the distal radioulnar joint (DRUJ) results in the head of the ulna dislocating dorsally. This can be seen as a prominent painful bony lump on the dorsum of the wrist. A classic examination test was to push the ulnar head down, only to feel it pop back up again dorsally. This was known as the piano key test. It is painful for the patient and not recommended! Treatment involves resection of the prominent ulnar head or replacement with a DRUJ arthroplasty.
- **MCP joint instability** – attenuation of the ligaments around the metacarpophalangeal joints results in drift in an ulnar direction of the metacarpals. The pull of the extensor tendons then becomes off-centre, causing them to act as bowstrings, exaggerating the deformity further. Eventually the MCP joints may dislocate. Early cases may be treated with soft tissue rebalancing procedures, more severe cases by replacing the joints with silicone spacers (Swanson arthroplasty).

- **Swan-neck and Boutonnière deformities** – the extensor tendons have a complex configuration in the fingers. Understanding the anatomy is important when considering the effect of RA. Rupture of the terminal slip of the extensor tendon at the distal interphalangeal joint (DIPJ) or rupture of the volar plate at the proximal interphalangeal joint (PIPJ) results in flexion of the DIPJ and hyperextension of the PIPJ due to increased tension in the tendon. This is a swan-neck deformity. Conversely, attenuation of the central extensor slip at the PIPJ combined with subluxation of the lateral bands over the PIPJ results in hyperextension of the DIPJ and flexion of the PIPJ. This is a Boutonnière deformity. Treatment involves splinting, reconstruction of the damaged structures or fusion of the joints.
- **Z-thumb** – similar to deformities seen in the fingers, the tendons and ligaments around the thumb may rupture. A variety of deformities may occur, but classically the MCP joint flexes and the interphalangeal joint hyperextends. Treatment consists of splints or fusion of selected joints.

Psoriatic arthritis

Also known as arthritis mutilans, extensive destruction of the joints causes very severe deformities in the hands. The fingers have a sausage-like appearance and X-rays show erosion of the phalanges resembling a 'pencil-in-cup'. Examine for scaly skin plaques. Sometimes the hands are affected before skin lesions are seen. The mainstay of treatment is medical but surgery has a role to play in fusion of badly affected joints.

Osteoarthritic wrist

Less common than RA in the wrist, osteoarthritis (OA) usually results from previous fractures of the radius or scaphoid or traumatic disruption of the ligaments that hold the carpal bones together.

Symptoms include pain, stiffness and limitation of movement, especially in extension. Ask about previous injuries when taking a history.

In contrast to RA, OA patients typically have much higher demands and want to return to manual activities, and treatment options reflect this. Options include:

- **Analgesia, physiotherapy and activity modification**.
- **Splinting** – either at night or for specific activities.
- **Selective arthrodesis** (fusion) of affected carpal bones – if arthritis is limited to only a few bones in the wrist, they can be fused. This abolishes pain with minimal restriction of movement.
- **Proximal row carpectomy** – the proximal row of the carpal bones (scaphoid, lunate, triquetrum) are excised and the wrist splinted for 6 weeks to allow scar tissue to fill the gap. Allows more movement than total wrist arthrodesis.
- **Total wrist arthrodesis** – fusion using a plate from the radius to the middle finger metacarpal – abolishes all movement in the wrist but reliably effective at relieving pain, whilst maintaining grip strength. Ideal for the young manual worker.
- **Wrist replacement** (wrist arthroplasty) is not recommended in high-demand or young patients due to rapid failure of the implants if subjected to excessive loading.

Wrist and hand 2

Figure 19.1   Carpal tunnel syndrome
(a) The carpal tunnel

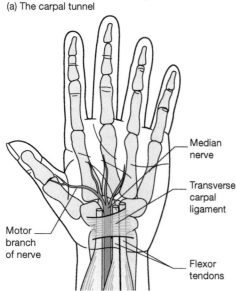

Median
nerve

Transverse
carpal
ligament

Motor
branch
of nerve

Flexor
tendons

(b) Carpal tunnel cross section. Note nine tendons and one nerve run through the tunnel

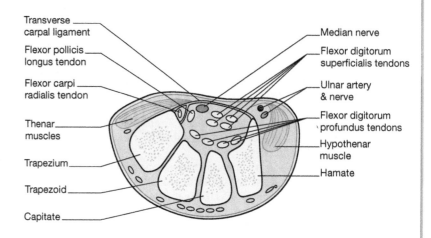

Transverse
carpal ligament

Flexor pollicis
longus tendon

Flexor carpi
radialis tendon

Thenar
muscles

Trapezium

Trapezoid

Capitate

Median nerve

Flexor digitorum
superficialis tendons

Ulnar artery
& nerve

Flexor digitorum
profundus tendons

Hypothenar
muscle

Hamate

(c) Sensory distribution of the median nerve

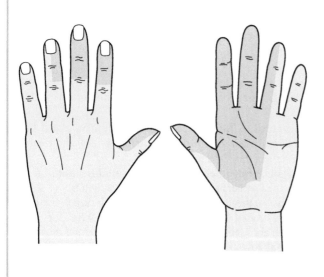

Figure 19.2   Other sites of median nerve compression

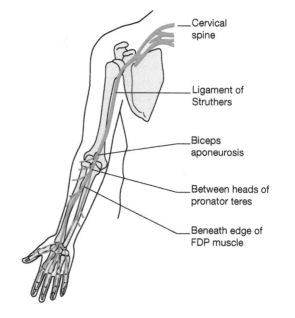

Cervical
spine

Ligament of
Struthers

Biceps
aponeurosis

Between heads of
pronator teres

Beneath edge of
FDP muscle

Carpal tunnel syndrome

Carpal tunnel syndrome is compression of the median nerve within the carpal tunnel and is the commonest peripheral compression neuropathy.

Relevant anatomy

The boundaries of the carpal tunnel are:
- **Radial**: scaphoid tubercle and trapezium.
- **Ulnar**: hook of hamate and pisiform.
- **Floor**: carpal bones and ligaments.
- **Roof**: transverse carpal ligament.
  The contents of the carpal tunnel are:
- median nerve;
- flexor pollicis longus (FPL) tendon;
- four flexor digitorum profundus tendons;
- four flexor digitorum superficialis tendons.
  The median nerve supplies:
- sensation to volar aspect of thumb, index, middle and half of ring fingers;
- motor to lateral two lumbricals, opponens pollicis, abductor pollicis, flexor pollicis brevis (LOAF).

Symptoms

Risk factors for development of carpal tunnel syndrome include pregnancy, diabetes, obesity, rheumatoid arthritis (RA; synovitis within tunnel) and malunion of distal radius fractures.

Typically patients complain of pain and paraesthesia in the thumb, index and middle fingers, worse after activity or at night. In severe or longstanding cases the muscles supplied by the median nerve become denervated resulting in weakness of thumb movements (especially abduction) and wasting of the thenar eminence.

Note that sensation to the lateral half of the palm is supplied by the palmar cutaneous branch of the median nerve, given off before the median nerve enters the carpal tunnel. This branch is therefore not affected by carpal tunnel syndrome.

Treatment

First-line treatment is activity modification and splints to wear at night. Splinting the wrist in neutral reduces pressure within the carpal tunnel.

Steroid injections into the carpal tunnel may be attempted but usually only offer temporary relief. They are a good option in pregnancy when the condition is transient and surgery is best avoided.

Surgical decompression represents the best long-term treatment option. This may be performed under local anaesthetic as a day case. The skin and fat are incised, avoiding the radially-positioned palmar cutaneous branch. The transverse carpal ligament is carefully divided.

It should be noted that the motor branch of the median nerve, also known as the recurrent motor branch, is usually given off just distal to the carpal tunnel, but in some individuals may branch within the carpal tunnel and penetrate the transverse carpal ligament, or rarely arise proximal to the transverse carpal ligament. The ligament should therefore be divided under direct vision.

Once the ligament is completely divided, the skin can be closed with interrupted sutures without tension. A bulky dressing is applied, which the patient reduces after 48 hours. The wound should be kept clean and dry until sutures are removed at around 12 days.

Complications of surgery

The usual complications of infection, bleeding and nerve damage may occur. Provided the surgery is performed carefully and wound care is adequate these should be uncommon. Failure to improve symptoms may represent incomplete division of the transverse carpal ligament. The commonest site for this is proximally. If the proximal extent of the ligament is visualised during surgery, this complication can be avoided. Persistent failure to improve should prompt investigation for sites of median nerve compression other than at the wrist.

Other sites of median nerve compression

Although the carpal tunnel is the commonest site for the median nerve to be compressed, it may be trapped anywhere along its course.
- **Cervical spine** – C5-T1 radiculopathy may mimic median nerve compression. The spine should always be examined.
- **Ligament of Struthers** – a rare variant of normal, some individuals have an abnormal spur of bone arising from the humerus called the supracondylar process. This is connected to the medial epicondyle of the humerus by a band of fibrous tissue called the ligament of Struthers (not to be confused with the arcade of Struthers which may trap the ulnar nerve!). The median nerve runs between the ligament and the distal humerus and may become trapped here.
- **Bicipital aponeurosis** – the biceps muscle sends a broad fibrous band into the forearm, properly known as the *lacertus fibrosis*. The nerve runs beneath it and may be trapped when the elbow is flexed and the forearm supinated.
- **Between the two heads of pronator teres** – symptoms occur in maximal pronation.
- **Beneath the proximal edge of flexor digitorum superficialis (FDS)** – rarely the proximal edge of FDS may trap the nerve against the radius just distal to the elbow.

Ulnar nerve neuropathy at the wrist

Much less common than carpal tunnel syndrome, the ulnar nerve may be compressed within Guyon's canal. This is a tight space bounded by the hook of hamate and pisiform and the fibrous arcade that connects these two bones, the volar carpal ligament.

Symptoms include sensory loss on the ulnar border of the palm and motor loss to the intrinsic muscles of the hand. Sensation to the dorsal aspect of the hand is spared because the dorsal cutaneous branch of the ulnar nerve arises proximal to Guyon's canal.

The commonest cause of compression is a ganglion arising from the carpal joints, although it may also occur following fracture of the hook of hamate or in association with long-term use of vibrating power tools.

Following MRI or ultrasound to confirm the site of compression, treatment is surgical decompression.

Compression of the ulnar nerve in Guyon's canal is much rarer than compression in the cubital tunnel at the elbow, discussed in Chapter 17.

20 Wrist and hand 3

Figure 20.1   Upper limb wrist and hand
(a) X-ray showing osteoarthritis of the first CMC joint. The left hand is most symptomatic. Note loss of joint space, osteophytes and subluxation

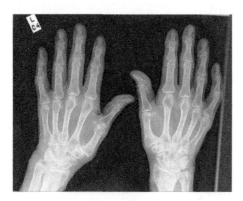

(b) Clinical appearance of first CMC OA

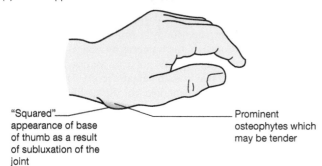

"Squared" appearance of base of thumb as a result of subluxation of the joint

Prominent osteophytes which may be tender

Figure 20.3
(a) Flexor tendons run through a system of pulleys. There are five 'annular' pulleys and three 'cruciform' pulleys

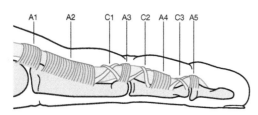

A1   A2   C1 A3 C2 A4 C3 A5

(b) Narrowing of the pulleys and formation of a nodule in the tendon results in triggering when the finger is flexed

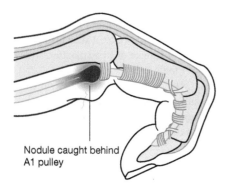

Nodule caught behind A1 pulley

Figure 20.2   Dupuytrens

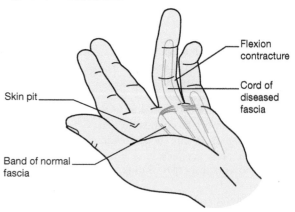

Flexion contracture

Cord of diseased fascia

Skin pit

Band of normal fascia

Figure 20.4
(a) The tendons of EPB and APL run through a tunnel just proximal to the radial styloid. In De Quervain's disease inflammation and narrowing of the tunnel results in pain

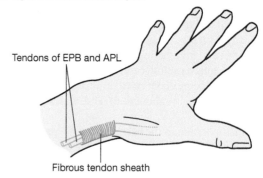

Tendons of EPB and APL

Fibrous tendon sheath

(b) Finkelstein's manoeuvre reproduces symptoms

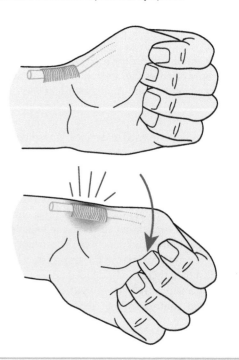

Trauma and Orthopaedics at a Glance, First Edition. Henry Willmott.
© 2016 John Wiley & Sons, Ltd. Published 2016 by John Wiley & Sons, Ltd. Companion website: www.ataglanceseries.com/TandO

First carpometacarpal osteoarthritis

The joint at the base of the thumb, the first carpometacarpal joint (1st CMC), is subjected to great force during grip, yet has a small surface area, making this joint susceptible to osteoarthritis (OA). Patients are typically elderly women, although young labourers may also be affected.

Symptoms include pain and weakness of grip. The thumb base develops a 'squared-off' appearance as osteophytes develop, the ligaments stretch and the joint becomes unstable.

Treatment options

- **Analgesia and splinting** in the first instance. Steroid injections offer temporary respite. Surgical options include:
- **Arthrodesis (fusion) of the joint** – a good option for young labourers as grip strength is maintained.
- **Replacement of the joint** with a silicone spacer or other prosthetic material. Although popular in the past, results have proven to be poor due to disintegration of the implant and resulting painful synovitis. This technique has largely been abandoned.
- **Excision of the trapezium: 'trapezectomy'** – simply excising the trapezium at the base of the thumb alleviates pain and has been proven to be a very effective treatment. The hand is put into plaster for several weeks after surgery, allowing scar tissue to form and fill the gap from where the trapezium was removed. The thumb may shorten as the metacarpal collapses to fill the gap. Some surgeons advocate augmenting trapezectomy with a ligament reconstruction to avoid this, although it does not improve functional results.

Dupuytren's disease

Dupuytren's disease is a benign condition in which the normal **fascial bands** in the palm and fingers contract to produce progressive contractures. Normal fibroblasts become replaced with **myofibroblasts**, which have a contractile component and lay down layers of collagen. This abnormal tissue is known as **cords**.

The disease is twice as common in men than women, with peak incidence in the 5–6th decades. Diabetes, alcoholism, HIV and anticonvulsive medication are all risk factors. The disease is almost unique to white populations. Inheritance is autosomal dominant with a link to Scandinavian ancestry. No link to occupation or trauma has been demonstrated.

Most cases are limited to the palm and fingers, but in severe cases, known as **Dupuytren's diathesis**, cords may form in the plantar fascia of the sole (**Ledderhose disease**), the knuckles (**Garrod's pads**) or the penis (**Peyronie's disease**).

Patients develop palpable cords within the palm, typically starting at the base of the ring finger. Small indentations known as skin pits may form. As the disease progresses the patient loses the ability to extend the metacarpophalangeal joint (MCPJ) and then the proximal interphalangeal joint (PIPJ). The distal interphalangeal joint (DIPJ) is never affected.

On examination feel the palm for cords and comment on skin pitting. Each joint in the hand should be examined in turn to assess for contracture and range of movement. Inspect the knuckles and ask if the patient has involvement of the feet. Intervention may be considered with MCPJ contractures exceeding 40° or PIPJ contractures exceeding 10°. As a rough guide, this correlates with an inability to lay the palm flat on a tabletop. If surgery is planned check the function of each digital nerve as they may be damaged intraoperatively.

Treatment options

- **Splinting** – there is little evidence that this is effective.
- **Percutaneous needle fasciotomy** – under local anaesthetic, a hypodermic needle is used to break down cords in the palm. A good option for patients with early disease, but risk to the nerves and arteries is high.
- **Collagenase injection** – this is a relatively new treatment in which an enzyme is injected into the cords to degrade collagen. The patient returns 24 hours later to have the finger manipulated. There is a risk of tendon rupture, and this treatment is not widely accepted at present.
- **Partial fasciectomy** – the most common method of treatment in which the cords are exposed through long incisions, nerves and arteries identified and diseased tissue carefully removed. In severe cases, it may prove impossible to close the skin after the contracture is corrected. In the palm the wound may be left open to heal by secondary intention but in the fingers full-thickness skin grafts may be needed. Recurrence occurs in up to 50% of cases.

Trigger finger

The tendons of flexor digitorum superficialis (FDS) and flexor digitorum profundus (FDP run through a system of pulleys on the palmar side of the fingers. The pulleys keep the tendons closely apposed to the bones and prevent bow-stringing when the fingers are flexed. Collectively the pulleys are known as the flexor sheath.

In trigger finger, the flexor sheath becomes narrowed and the normal gliding motion of the tendons is restricted. This results in the formation of an inflammatory nodule within the tendon itself. The tightness of the flexor sheath combined with the tendon nodule results in the tendon catching and getting stuck at the mouth of the flexor sheath. The patient may overcome this with a sudden click, which is detected as a painful 'triggering' sensation. In severe cases the patient may be unable to release the stuck tendon.

Why the flexor sheath should become narrowed is unclear. It is more common in diabetics and patients with rheumatoid arthritis. Most cases are idiopathic.

Treatment options

- **Steroid injection** into the flexor sheath may reduce swelling and alleviate the triggering phenomenon. Repeat injections may be needed and recurrence is common.
- **Surgical release of the first pulley**: under local anaesthetic the mouth of the flexor sheath can be opened with a longitudinal slit in the first pulley. This is usually a permanent solution.

de Quervain's disease

This is inflammation and narrowing of the first dorsal compartment of the wrist, the fascial tunnel through which the tendons of extensor pollicis brevis (EPB) and abductor pollicis longus (APL) run.

Patients complain of pain over the radial styloid, which is exacerbated by wrist movement. It may be caused by repetitive sprain or overuse, or may be idiopathic. It is often seen in postpartum women.

Pain may be reproduced by **Finkelstein's manoeuvre**, which is forced ulnar deviation of the wrist with the thumb tucked in the palm.

Treatment consists of splinting and activity modification, augmented by steroid injections. Recalcitrant cases may require surgical release of the tendon sheath.

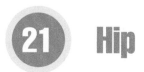

21 Hip

Figure 21.1   AP pelvis x-ray demonstrating early OA of both hips

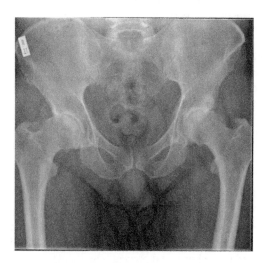

Figure 21.2   AP pelvis x-ray demonstrating advanced OA of the right hip

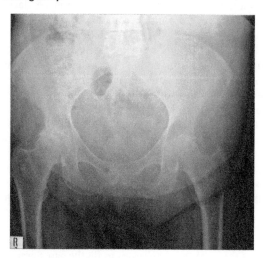

Figure 21.3   Osteonecrosis of the hip

(a) AP pelvis x-ray demonstrating osteonecrosis of the right hip. Note the dense sclerotic bone. The subchondral bone has died and collapsed resulting in a radioleucent line beneath the articular surface: The 'crescent sign'

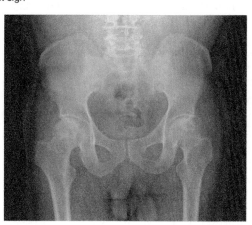

(b) Sagittal STIR MRI sequence demonstrating osteonecrosis affecting the head of the right femur

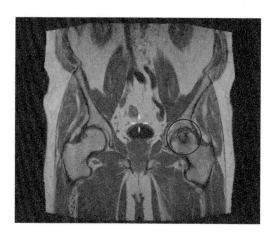

Trauma and Orthopaedics at a Glance, First Edition. Henry Willmott.
© 2016 John Wiley & Sons, Ltd. Published 2016 by John Wiley & Sons, Ltd. Companion website: www.ataglanceseries.com/TandO

Hip arthritis

One of the most common conditions treated by orthopaedic surgeons, hip arthritis affects many older people. Loss of the cartilage of the hip joint results in pain and stiffness as the bony surfaces of the femoral head and the acetabulum come into contact.

Risk factors

Hip arthritis is more commonly seen in patients over 50. Most cases are idiopathic 'wear and tear', but in some patients there may be a predisposing factor:

- **Inflammatory arthritis** (RA, SLE, psoriatic arthritis) – systemic comditions that may affect multiple joints.
- **Osteonecrosis** – discussed below, results in collapse of the femoral head.
- **Previous septic arthritis** – enzymes produced by bacterial infection destroy cartilage. Active infection is a contraindication to joint replacement.
- **Abnormal hip shape** – hip dysplasia, old slipped capital femoral epiphysis (SCFE), femoroacetabular impingement and old Perthes' disease are developmental conditions that alter the shape of the 'ball-and-socket' joint, resulting in increased wear. Patients may develop osteoarthritis (OA) in their third or fourth decade.

Signs and symptoms

- **Pain:** Patients complain of groin, buttock or thigh pain. Initially pain is only present with movement but eventually may become constant, even preventing sleep at night.
- **Stiffness:** typically patients are unable to cross their legs and getting out of a low chair or car is difficult
- **Limp:** a combination of pain, stiffness and weak muscles around the hip results in a limp and the classic Trendelenburg gait, which may resemble a drunken sailor's lurch.

Examination

- **Gait** assessment and comment on stick or frame.
- **Trendelenburg test** whilst the patient is standing to assess for weak abductors.
- **Range of movement** – first do Thomas' test to exclude fixed flexion deformity, then assess all movements compared to the contralateral side: flexion, extension, abduction and adduction, internal and external rotation with the hip extended and in flexion.
- **Leg length** – erosion of the acetabulum may cause true shortening; fixed abduction contracture may cause apparent shortening.
- **Neurovascular examination** of the legs (feel for pulses and sensation) and brief assessment of lumbar spine and the knee.

Differential diagnosis

- **Spine:** mechanical back pain may cause buttock or groin pain. Radiculopathy (root impingement) may cause shooting pains down the back of the leg, typically extending below the knee.
- **Knee:** knee pathology may cause thigh pain or limping.
- **Tumour:** primary bone tumours are rare, bony metastases are very common! Weight loss, history of cancer (especially breast and prostate), constant pain or night pain are red flags. Obtain full length femoral X-rays or a bone scan if in doubt.
- **Infection:** septic arthritis or osteomyelitis, although history is usually short and patients systemically unwell.
- **Stress fracture** of the femoral neck may be seen in runners; subtrochanteric fractures occur in elderly patients on bisphosphonates due to inhibition of bone remodelling. Demonstrated on X-ray or MRI.
- **Greater trochanteric bursitis:** inflammation of the bursa between the iliotibial band and the greater trochanter may cause sharp localised pain. Patients typically cannot lie on their side. MRI demonstrates it well. Steroid and local anaesthetic injection may be helpful, physiotherapy for long-term treatment.

Investigations

- **X-rays** – AP pelvis and lateral of the affected hip. Look for the LOSS signs. Comment on leg length and the position of the femoral head in the acetabulum. The lumbar spine, full-length femur and knee may also need X-rays.
- **Bloods** – routine pre-op bloods if surgery is planned, C-reactive protein (CRP)/erythrocyte sedimentation rate (ESR) and rheumatoid factor (RhF)/antinuclear antibodies (ANA) if inflammatory arthritis suspected.
- **CT/MRI** – CT is good at assessing bone loss if the acetabulum is severely eroded. MRI assesses soft tissues around the hip as well as the state of the cartilage if the diagnosis is not clear.

Treatment options

- Weight loss, analgesia, activity modification.
- Physiotherapy and the use of a stick.
- Total hip replacement – discussed in Chapter 22.

Osteonecrosis (avascular necrosis)

Loss of the blood supply to bone is known as osteonecrosis. All joints can be affected but the femoral head is at risk because its blood supply is retrograde and tenuous (see Chapter 43).

Causes of femoral head osteonecrosis

- **Idiopathic** – most cases.
- **Trauma** – intracapsular neck of femur fractures disrupt the retinacular blood vessels that supply blood to the femoral head.
- **Steroids** – alterations in fat metabolism result in lipid globules in the blood, which block arterioles.
- **Long-term alcohol use**.
- **Haemoglobinopathies** (e.g. sickle-cell anaemia).
- **'The bends'** – divers ascending too quickly develop nitrogen bubbles in the blood, which may block arterioles.

Pathophysiology

Bone just below the cartilage (subchondral bone) is the most susceptible to die if the blood supply is interrupted. Initially the patient complains of pain in the hip, but X-rays appear normal. After a period of 3–6 months, dead subchondral bone appears dense on X-ray. Several weeks thereafter, the dead bone is resorbed and a linear lucency develops. This is known as the crescent sign.

If the patient continues weightbearing, the femoral head collapses, losing its spherical shape and resulting in secondary osteoarthritis.

Treatment

Initially make the patient non-weightbearing to prevent femoral head collapse. Physiotherapy maintains range of movement.

- **Core decompression:** in early cases, before the crescent sign has appeared or the head has collapsed, drilling a tunnel up the femoral neck and into the head relieves pressure, improves blood flow and may stimulate bone healing. Results are not guaranteed.
- **Total hip replacement:** once the head has collapsed, this is the only surgical option.

22 Hip replacement

Figure 22.1 Hip resurfacing

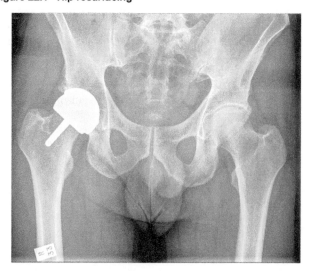

Figure 22.2 Total hip replacement
The stem has been cemented into the femur. The acetabulum is uncemented and held by impaction and a single screw for added stability. Note the skin clips in this patient, indicating that the x-ray was taken in the immediate post-operative period

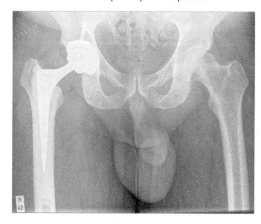

Figure 22.3 Uncemented THR
The surface of the components is rough so that it 'grips' the bone and encourages bone integration

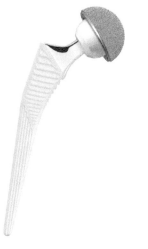

"Reproduced by permission of DePuySynthes International Ltd"

Figure 22.4 Cemented stem THR with uncemented acetabulum
Note that in contrast to the uncemented stem, the surface of the cemented stem is smooth and shiny

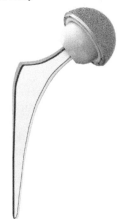

"Reproduced by permission of DePuySynthes International Ltd"

Figure 22.5 Dislocated THR
The patient was climbing into the bath when he felt sudden pain in his right hip and fell to the floor. The hip is dislocated. The acetabular component has been malpositioned such that the risk of dislocation is increased. The patient underwent revision hip replacement in order to prevent repeat dislocation

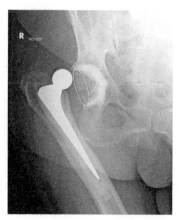

Trauma and Orthopaedics at a Glance, First Edition. Henry Willmott.
© 2016 John Wiley & Sons, Ltd. Published 2016 by John Wiley & Sons, Ltd. Companion website: www.ataglanceseries.com/TandO

The role of total hip replacement

One of the most commonly performed orthopaedic procedures, total hip replacement (THR) is indicated for the treatment of osteoarthritis of the hip when conservative treatment has failed and symptoms are severe enough to warrant surgery.

Types of hip replacement

Broadly speaking there are three main types:

- **Total hip replacement** – the femoral head is replaced with a prosthetic ball and the acetabulum is relined with a prosthetic cup.
- **Resurfacing** – a technique in which the patient's femoral head is preserved and resurfaced with a metal shell. The acetabulum is relined in the same way as a THR. Originally developed for younger patients, the preservation of bone made potential future revision easier. Unfortunately the system was very sensitive to errors of placement, and even small deviations from perfect positioning resulted in femoral neck fracture, rapid wear of bearings and generation of excess metal debris. As a result failure rates were high and this technique has largely fallen out of favour.
- **Hemi-arthroplasty** – replacement of the femoral head only, without addressing the acetabulum. Used for treatment of femoral neck fractures (see Chapter 44).

Cemented vs uncemented

The prosthesis may be secured to the bone using bone cement. Bone cement is a polymer called polymethylmethacrylate. It acts as a grout and is injected into the femoral canal under pressure to ensure it becomes deeply embedded into the prepared bone surface. Pressurisation may have the unintended effect of forcing fat out of the marrow and into the blood stream, which may cause intraoperative hypotension and cardiovascular collapse during the operation.

Alternatively an uncemented prosthesis may be used. These prostheses are coated in hydroxyapatite (the same chemical compound of calcium and phosphate as found in bone) and have a roughened surface to encourage bone to integrate with the prosthesis, creating a 'biological' bond. Theoretically this is longer lasting than cement and avoids the issues associated with fat embolism. However, the tight fit required may result in fractures of the femur or pelvis occurring as the prosthesis is implanted.

Bearing surfaces

The interface between the ball of the femoral head and the cup of the acetabulum is known as the bearing. The bearing carries significant load and must be low friction and hard wearing. If the bearing wears out, the hip has to be revised. There are a number of different bearing materials available, each with pros and cons.

- **Polyethylene** – used in the acetabulum, it is cheap and low friction. Modern polyethylenes are fairly hard wearing but do wear out with time. As they wear, they produce debris in the form of polyethylene particles ranging from 0.1 to 10 microns in size. These small particles are the same size as bacteria, and this similarity stimulates white blood cells to produce inflammatory cytokines. The cytokines in turn stimulate osteoclasts to resorb bone around the prosthesis, resulting in loosening and premature failure of the implant. This process is called osteolysis.
- **Metal** – used to make femoral heads for many years, metal is cheap and hard wearing, working well with polyethylene acetabular liners. Recently metal was used as the acetabular bearing, but this resulted in large amounts of metal wear debris being produced.

This caused problems with systemic toxicity and local inflammation and has now been discontinued.

- **Ceramic** – very hard wearing and extremely low friction, this is a good material for both acetabular liners and femoral heads. It is so hard that there is virtually no wear, making it a good option for young patients. It is expensive to produce. It is brittle and may fracture if exposed to sudden shock loading. Rarely, ceramic-on-ceramic bearings can produce a squeaking noise on movement.

Complications of THR

- **Nerve injury** – the sciatic nerve is particularly at risk resulting in foot drop and numbness in the foot. Common causes include traction on the nerve or compression by retractor placement.
- **Bleeding** – average blood loss is 250 mL, but a proportion of patients lose more and require blood transfusion.
- **Deep vein thrombosis (DVT)/pulmonary embolism (PE)** – without prophylactic blood-thinning, deep vein thrombosis (DVT) is common after THR. Chemical and mechanical thromboprophylaxis should be used routinely.
- **Infection** – this is a major problem and all measures are taken to avoid it, including a clean air supply in theatre, antibiotic-loaded cement and perioperative antibiotics. If the prosthesis becomes infected, a two-stage revision may be indicated in which the hip is removed and the patient given antibiotics for 6 weeks before a new prosthesis is implanted.
- **Dislocation** – may occur if the soft tissues are not balanced or the prosthesis is malpositioned intraoperatively. Precautions including avoidance of crossing legs, bending over and sitting in low chairs, which are implemented by the physiotherapists postoperatively.
- **Leg length discrepancy** – if the acetabulum has been severely eroded or the hip is an abnormal shape, leg length differences are more common. Careful preoperative planning helps avoid this. Up to 15 mm difference is usually well tolerated by the patient.

Investigation of the painful THR

- **Infection** – this is the first diagnosis to exclude. Infection may occur many years after the surgery. It may be due to bacteria introduced at the time of surgery, or haematogenous spread of bacteria in conjunction with an infection elsewhere in the body, such as a dental abscess. Check C-reactive protein (CRP)/erythrocyte sedimentation rate (ESR) and get a bone scan, which will show increased uptake around the prosthesis.
- **Loosening** – may be due to polyethylene debris osteolysis or infection. X-ray signs of loosening include a lucent line around the prosthesis or migration of the prosthesis on serial views.
- **Fracture** – may occur intraoperatively, especially with uncemented implants, or postoperatively following a fall. If the femoral stem is loose it needs to be revised; if it remains fixed in the femur, cables and a plate can be used to reconstruct the bone around the stem.
- **Other diagnoses** – if a patient's pain never got better after a THR, was the original diagnosis correct? Check the spine; consider other causes of pain in the groin, buttock and thigh.

National Joint Registry

Since 2007, all hip and knee replacements have been recorded on a national database. Shoulder, elbow and ankle replacements are now also included. This allows monitoring of failure rates, early detection of failing implants and production of statistics analysing individual surgeon's outcomes.

23 Knee 1

Figure 23.1 Varus knee osteoarthritis
Note loss of the medial joint space, subchondral sclerosis, osteophytes. The knee is in varus alignment

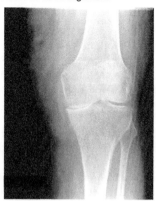

Figure 23.2 X-ray of unicompartmental knee replacement
Only the medial compartment has been resurfaced and normal anatomical alignment has been restored

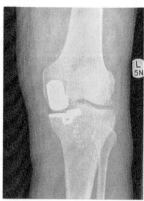

Figure 23.3 X-ray of total knee replacement
(a) AP view; (b) Lateral view

(a)

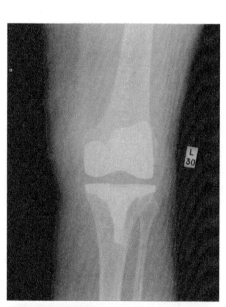

(b)

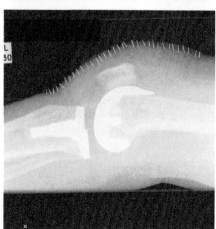

Figure 23.4 Loosening in a TKR
A: Wear of the plastic bearing of the TKR results in the production of small wear particles which are roughly the same size as bacteria.
B: Macrophages phagocytose the wear particles.
C: Macrophages produce cytokines and intracellular signalling molecules. This results in recruitment of more macrophages and lymphocytes which causes swelling and synovitis.
D: The cytokines activate osteoclast precursors which differentiate into active osteoclasts.
E: Osteoclasts resorb bone around the implant, resulting in a leucent line on x-rays, cysts and loosening of the component.

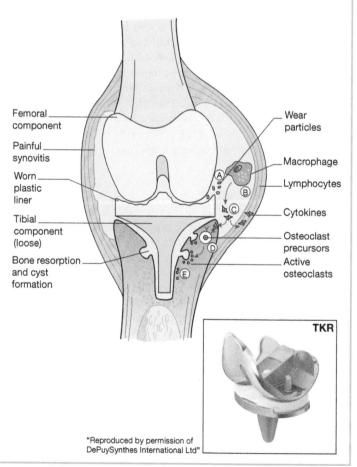

Femoral component
Painful synovitis
Worn plastic liner
Tibial component (loose)
Bone resorption and cyst formation

Wear particles
Macrophage
Lymphocytes
Cytokines
Osteoclast precursors
Active osteoclasts

TKR

Trauma and Orthopaedics at a Glance, First Edition. Henry Willmott.
© 2016 John Wiley & Sons, Ltd. Published 2016 by John Wiley & Sons, Ltd. Companion website: www.ataglanceseries.com/TandO

The knee

The knee joint comprises the interface of three bones: the femur, the tibia and the patella. The femur has two condyles and anteriorly a notch called the trochlea, in which the patella slides as the knee flexes. The patella is a sesamoid bone with the quadriceps tendon above and the patellar tendon below. The proximal end of the tibia is covered with two fibrocartilaginous structures, the menisci. The joint is stabilised by anterior and posterior cruciate ligaments at the centre of the joint, and a medial and lateral collateral ligament either side.

Although the knee has only one joint cavity anatomically, functionally it is helpful to consider the knee as three compartments:
- the patellofemoral compartment – between trochlea and patella;
- the medial compartment – between medial femoral condyle and medial tibial plateau;
- the lateral compartment – between lateral femoral condyle and lateral tibial plateau.

Thinking of the knee in this way facilitates treatment decision-making.

Knee osteoarthritis

As in other synovial joints, osteoarthritis (OA) may be idiopathic (wear and tear) or secondary to trauma or infection.

Symptoms are pain, stiffness, crepitus and loss of movement. X-ray findings include loss of joint space, formation of osteophytes, subchondral sclerosis and cysts (remembered by the mnemonic LOSS), and in severe cases, loss of the normal anatomical alignment of the limb.

Clinically the patient may demonstrate swelling, stiffness – especially loss of extension – and deformity in the form of malalignment. Malalignment may be varus (bow-legged) or valgus (knock-kneed) depending on whether the OA affects either the medial or lateral compartments, respectively. Varus OA is the commonest form. It is easiest to demonstrate malalignment with the patient standing and viewed from behind.

Treatment

Initially conservative treatment should include weight loss, activity modification and physiotherapy to improve strength, range of movement and proprioception. Failure of these measures may be an indication for surgery. There are a number of surgical options.

Knee arthroscopy

Although traditionally it was thought that washing the knee out by means of an arthroscopy improved symptoms, this has not been borne out by clinical trials. Any improvement in symptoms is short-lived, and this procedure is not recommended by the National Institute for Health and Care Excellence (NICE) as a treatment for OA. It may have a role in the debridement of degenerate meniscal tears, which cause mechanical symptoms in selected young patients.

Patellofemoral joint replacement

Osteoarthritis of the patellofemoral joint (PFJ) causes anterior knee pain, which is worse coming down stairs: loading the knee in the flexed position generates high forces through the PFJ. If arthritis involves only the PFJ, selective replacement of this part of the joint may be indicated. The procedure is usually performed in younger patients, in whom a total knee replacement would not be expected to last their lifetime. Failure and revision rates of patellofemoral replacements are high because large areas of the knee are left untreated, which allows OA to progress.

High tibial osteotomy

Some young, active patients have OA limited to the medial compartment resulting in varus malalignment of the limb. The malalignment may be corrected by cutting and realigning the tibia. Correcting the axis of the limb in this way reduces force transmission through the diseased part of the knee and reduces pain. It delays the need for a total knee replacement by up to 10 years in 50% of cases.

Unicompartmental knee replacement

If OA affects just the medial or lateral compartment, half the knee can be replaced. This is known as a unicompartmental knee replacement. The patient must not have significant stiffness or deformity and the cruciate ligaments must be intact. It is a difficult procedure to get right, and only a few patients fit the criteria. Revision rates are high.

Total knee replacement (TKR)

Replacement of the whole joint is the most commonly performed surgical procedure for tricompartmental OA of the knee. The knee is opened anteriorly and the patella flipped over in a lateral direction to allow access to the joint. The end of the femur is cut with a cutting-block and a metal prosthesis cemented into position. The tibia is cut using a jig to realign the axis of the limb. A metal and plastic prosthesis is cemented in place. The underside of the patella may also be resurfaced with a plastic button.

A TKR should improve range of movement, treat pain and restore the normal axis of the limb. It is vital that the collateral ligaments are preserved in order to maintain stability. The thickness of the plastic tibial component and the amount of bone resected from the femur and tibia may be varied in order to achieve stability of the knee in both flexion and extension. This process is known as balancing the flexion and extension gaps.

Complications of TKR: These include:
- **Infection** – as with all prosthetic joints, infection may be introduced at the time of surgery, develop in the wound in the immediate perioperative period, or be seeded years later by bacteraemia from another source. Presentation is pain, swelling, warmth and signs of sepsis. Aspiration of the joint allows an organism to be identified, but in contrast to a native joint, if an arthroplasty is in situ, do not aspirate in A&E or on the ward! It must be done in theatre under aseptic conditions! If the infection occurs within a few weeks of surgery, the joint may be saved by rapid return to theatre for debridement, washout and change of the plastic liner. If this fails or the patient presents late, the joint must be revised in two stages with a prolonged course of antibiotics.
- **Damage to nerves or blood vessels** – the tibial nerve, common peroneal nerve and popliteal artery are close to the back of the knee and may be damaged intraoperatively either by a saw blade or traction. Always check pulses, power and sensation in the foot when the spinal anaesthetic has worn off.
- **Dislocation of patella** – improper release of soft tissues or malpositioning of the implants may result in the patella dislocating.
- **Instability** – usually due to improper balancing or damage to the collaterals.
- **Wear and loosening** – just as in total hip replacement, in TKR the plastic bearing wears, generating debris that results in osteolysis and loosening. Studies show that more than 90% of TKRs survive for 15 years. A lucent line on X-ray, accompanied by pain and loss of stability, is an indication for revision although infection must be excluded first.

24 Knee 2

Figure 24.1 Meniscal tear

(a) Loading the knee in flexion causes painful clicking or locking

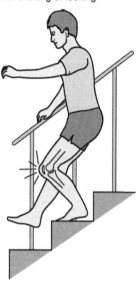

(b) Types of meniscal tears

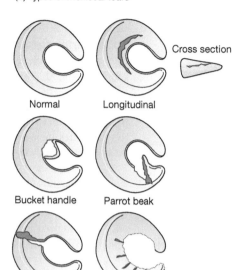

Normal

Longitudinal

Cross section

Bucket handle

Parrot beak

Radial

Degenerate

(c) MRI of meniscal tear. Sagittal STIR sequence showing increased signal in the posterior horn of the medial meniscus

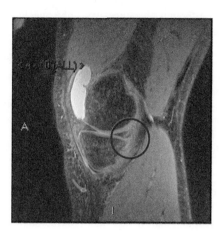

Figure 24.2 PLC injury

(a) Forcing the tibia backwards such as a dashboard impaction in a car crash my disrupt the PLC

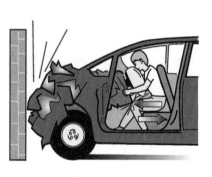

(b) Extreme twisting of the knee may disrupt the ACL. This may be combined with MCL or medial meniscus injury

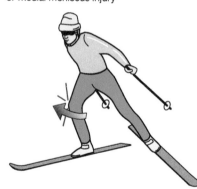

(c) Extreme varus or valgus force, such as a rugby tackle from the side, may disrupt the collateral ligaments

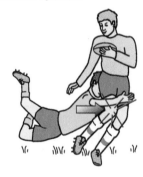

Meniscal tears

The structure and function of the menisci are discussed in Chapter 1. The most important function of the menisci is to bear load across the joint. Load bearing is greatest with the knee in the flexed position, with 90% of the load passing through the menisci in 90° flexion.

In a twisting injury the menisci may become torn, most commonly the medial meniscus. Adolescents or young adults are most commonly affected. Pain is localised to the joint line, worse when loading the knee in flexion, such as coming down stairs. Mechanical symptoms such as locking or catching are classic.

Examination findings include joint line tenderness and a small effusion. McMurray's test is a provocative test in which the knee is loaded and twisted in flexion producing a painful click.

In contrast to acute tears, chronic tears occur in older patients without a history of trauma. They are due to degeneration and osteoarthritis (OA).

Imaging should include an X-ray to exclude arthritis or fracture. MRI is the best modality to demonstrate a tear. There are various descriptive terms to describe tear morphology including bucket handle, parrot beak, longitudinal and radial.

Treatment is usually via arthroscopy:
- **Debridement:** trimming the torn edge back to a stable base. If large amounts of meniscus are removed, more force is transmitted to the cartilage, and the risk of OA in the future is increased.
- **Repair:** only the peripheral third of the meniscus has a blood supply. Certain tears in this region can heal if repaired. Indications for repair are non-degenerative longitudinal or bucket-handle tears within 5 mm of the periphery of the meniscus. Tears extending into the avascular central portion of the meniscus will not heal.

Ligament injuries

The knee has four important ligaments: medial and lateral collaterals and anterior and posterior cruciates. They stabilise the knee against varus/valgus, anterior/posterior translation and twisting.

Anterior cruciate ligament (ACL) tears

These occur with the twisting forces experienced by skiers and footballers. As the ligament ruptures, patients may hear a pop and the knee gives way. The ligament contains an artery, which bleeds into the knee when torn. This results in a large effusion developing within minutes. ACL ruptures may be associated with meniscal tears and medial collateral ligament (MCL) rupture, a combination of injuries known as the 'terrible triad'.

Diagnosis is based on the history and clinical examination. Disruption of the ACL results in a positive anterior drawer (excessive anterior translation of the tibia in 90° flexion), Lachman's test (excessive AP sloppiness in 30° flexion) and pivot-shift test (subluxation of the tibia with external rotation and valgus that reduces with a clunk on flexion). MRI is the best imaging modality.

Treatment of isolated ACL injury is initially conservative with specialist physiotherapy to train the quadriceps to stabilise the knee. If this fails and instability remains, ACL reconstruction may be carried out using a graft obtained from the patient's hamstrings or patellar tendon.

Posterior cruciate ligament (PCL) injuries

These occur when the tibia is forced backwards with the knee flexed. This occurs when a car occupant strikes the dashboard in a collision. PCL injuries are rare in isolation and may be associated with multiligamentous injury (see below). Treatment of isolated PCL injury is initially physiotherapy and bracing, but surgical reconstruction may be carried out.

Collateral ligament injuries

These occur when the knee is subjected to severe valgus or varus injury, such as being tackled from the side. Isolated injuries are commonly treated conservatively in a hinged brace, which stabilises the knee against varus/valgus stress.

Multiligamentous knee injury ('knee dislocation')

This is a serious limb-threatening injury. It takes a large amount of energy to dislocate the knee, and associated life-threatening injuries may coexist. The danger of a dislocated knee is that the popliteal artery may be damaged, resulting in limb ischaemia. Unstable knee dislocations should be stabilised initially with an external fixator and an arteriogram performed urgently. Reconstruction may be performed in stages and is technically demanding. Note that knee dislocation where the femur and tibia dislocate is not the same as the (much more benign) patellar dislocation, where the patella slips out of the trochlea.

Isolated osteochondral defects

Trauma to the knee may damage areas of cartilage. This is detectable on MRI. Left unchecked, osteoarthritis may develop. In young patients with a discrete area of cartilage damage, arthroscopy allows evaluation and treatment. Cartilage flaps may be debrided, and procedures carried out either to stimulate fibrocartilage formation, or transplant healthy cartilage from elsewhere in the joint (see Chapter 3).

The swollen knee

A common referral from A&E and GPs is an acutely swollen knee. The differential diagnosis includes:
- **Septic arthritis** – Bacteria may enter the joint by direct inoculation, from adjacent osteomyelitis or via haematogenous seeding. The joint is hot, swollen and erythematous and any movement is very painful. Aspirate may show pus or turbid fluid. Microscopy shows neutrophils and organisms may also be seen. Treatment is urgent wash-out of the joint in theatre. Antibiotics should be given only after an aspirate has been obtained.
- **Crystal arthropathy** – Gout is crystals of uric acid precipitating within the joint. Crystals are thin, needle-shaped and negatively birefringent on polarised light microscopy. The disease often also affects other joints, especially the first metatarsophalangeal joint (MTP) joint. It may be due to an idiopathic error in purine metabolism or to increased protein turnover in haemolytic anaemia or after chemotherapy. Pseudogout is a disorder in which calcium pyrophosphate crystals form. They are rhomboid and positively birefringent, and the condition tends to affect older people. X-rays of the knee may show calcification of the menisci known as chondrocalcinosis.
- **Haemarthrosis** – blood in the joint. Associated with trauma or spontaneous. May be due to coagulopathy or warfarin. If associated with trauma, consider ligamentous injury (especially ACL) or fracture. Fractured bone results in a mixture of blood and fat in the joint – a lipohaemarthrosis. Fat floats – it is less dense than blood – and this may be seen on X-ray as two distinct fluid levels. Aspirate reveals fat globules in the syringe.
- **Inflammatory arthropathy** – the commonest is rheumatoid arthritis (RA), but many other types exist. Onset is usually insidious, affecting multiple joints,. There may be a history of systemic illness such as inflammatory bowel disease. Check erythrocyte sedimentation rate (ESR), C-reactive protein (CRP), rheumatoid factor (RhF) and antinuclear antibodies (ANA).
- **Bursitis** – swelling outside the knee joint: prepatellar bursitis (housemaid's knee) or infrapatellar bursitis (parson's knee) are diagnosed by careful examination.

25 Foot and ankle

Figure 25.1 Osteoarthritis of the ankle

(a) X-ray showing ankle arthritis. Note loss of joint space and prominent osteophytes

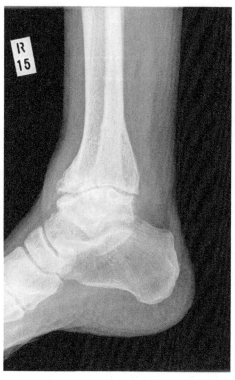

(b) X-ray of an ankle fusion. The joint surfaces have been resected and fixed with two screws. Plantar flexion and dorsiflexion are eliminated

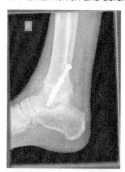

(c) X-ray of a total ankle replacement. Movement is maintained but in very active patients the bearing may wear out rapidly

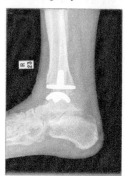

Figure 25.2 Tibialis posterior insufficiency

(a) Stage 2 tibialis posterior insufficiency. The hindfoot is in varus. The arches have collapsed. On the left, the 'too many toes sign' is seen, indicating excessive abduction of the forefoot
(b) The same patient when asked to stand on tiptoes. The heel stays in varus and she is unable to single stance heel raise

(a)   (b)

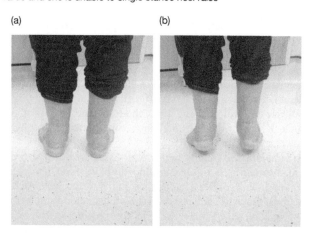

Figure 25.3 Hallux valgus

(a) Weight-bearing AP x-ray of the foot showing hallux valgus. The first metatarsal is in valgus, the first MTP joint is incongruent and there is a bunion
(b) Postoperative x-ray of the same patient showing a corrective osteotomy of the first metatarsal. The bunion has also been trimmed

(a)   (b)

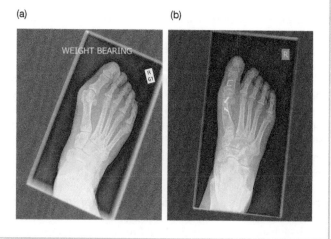

Trauma and Orthopaedics at a Glance, First Edition. Henry Willmott.
© 2016 John Wiley & Sons, Ltd. Published 2016 by John Wiley & Sons, Ltd. Companion website: www.ataglanceseries.com/TandO

Osteoarthritis

Osteoarthritis (OA) may affect any joint in the foot or ankle. It may be idiopathic or secondary to trauma. The symptoms vary according to which joint is affected:

Ankle arthritis limits dorsiflexion and plantarflexion. In maximal dorsiflexion, osteophytes on the anterior margin of the joint get trapped between the talus and the tibia, known as anterior impingement.

Subtalar arthritis results in pain when walking on uneven ground as the hindfoot tries to accommodate in varus/valgus.

Midfoot arthritis includes many joints – pain is commonly felt dorsally, exacerbated by walking. Patients may notice prominent osteophytes and collapse of the arch.

First metatarsophalangeal joint arthritis, also known as hallux rigidus, may be associated with a bunion. Pain is worse when standing on tiptoe and walking barefoot, as this is when movement of the joint is greatest.

Treatment: Treatment of OA includes:

- **Analgesia**.
- **Activity modification** – change occupation and style of footwear.
- **Orthotics** – insoles and stiff-soled shoes.
- **Target injection** – it is often hard to decide which joint is arthritic, especially in the midfoot. Injections of local anaesthetic and steroid, placed under X-ray guidance, offer short-term relief, and also guide the surgeon as to which joints are the most painful.
- **Arthroscopic debridement** – an option for the ankle and subtalar joint; removal of osteophytes and debridement of damaged cartilage may alleviate symptoms to some extent.
- **Arthrodesis** (fusion) – eliminating movement by removing any residual cartilage from the bone ends before rigidly fixing the joint with screws and/or plates to allow the joint to fuse. Non-union may occur in smokers or diabetics.
- **Joint replacement** – prosthetic ankle replacement allows movement to remain but complication rates are high. In very physically active patients, early failure of the implant may result.

Rheumatoid arthritis

In contrast to OA, soft-tissue attenuation is the main problem in rheumatoid arthritis (RA). Joints may become unstable, and in combination with bone erosion, may sublux or dislocate. The forefoot is often affected first, with dislocated metatarsophalangeal (MTP) joints and overlapping toes. The midfoot and hindfoot may also be involved.

Treatment starts with systemic disease control, anti-inflammatories and orthotics. Surgical intervention is usually in the form of fusion, as this will treat both instability and pain. Periarticular bone erosion and steroid-related osteoporosis can make this technically challenging. If significant deformity exists, the more proximal joints should be corrected first.

Tibialis posterior insufficiency

The tibialis posterior tendon runs round the posterior aspect of the medial malleolus and has insertions into all of the bones of the midfoot. The main insertion is into the navicular. It acts an inverter of the hindfoot and adductor of the forefoot. It also maintains the medial longitudinal arch of the foot.

The tendon has an area of relatively poor blood supply as it passes behind the medial malleolus. In middle age this section of the tendon may become degenerate and stretched or eventually rupture.

The result is pain and swelling behind the medial malleolus and eventually loss of the medial longitudinal arch, abduction of the forefoot and eversion (valgus) of the hindfoot. This is known as a planovalgus deformity. Classically patients are unable to stand on tiptoes (heel raise) and the abducted position of the forefoot leads to the 'too many toes' sign when viewed from behind.

Staging: Tibialis posterior insufficiency can be split into four stages, which determine the treatment.

Stage	Deformity	Heel raise	Arthritis
1	None. Pain/swelling behind medial malleolus	Yes	No
2	Flexible planovalgus	No	No
3	Rigid planovalgus	No	Subtalar
4	Rigid planovalgus	No	Subtalar and ankle

Treatment: This is determined by the stage of the disease:

Stage 1: insole, debridement of tendon.

Stage 2: because the planovalgus is flexible and correctable, the torn tibialis posterior tendon can be reconstructed by transferring flexor digitorum longus tendon into the navicular.

Stage 3: fusion of the subtalar, calcaneocuboid and talonavicular joints ('triple fusion').

Stage 4: triple fusion plus ankle fusion ('pantalar fusion') – which severely limits mobility.

Hallux valgus and hallux rigidus

Hallux valgus is medial deviation of the first metatarsal and lateral deviation of the proximal phalanx of the first toe. The prominent metatarsal head may form a painful bunion. It is more common in women and may be related to footwear.

Most cases can be treated simply with accommodative, wide-fitting shoes. If this fails and pain is present, surgical correction may be considered.

The objective of surgery is to realign the first metatarsal with the long axis of the foot. This may be achieved in a number of ways, depending on the severity of the deformity, but generally a corrective osteotomy of the first metatarsal is performed. This may be augmented with fusion of the first tarsometatarsal joint if it is hypermobile, and corrective osteotomy of the proximal phalanx if it is contributing to the deformity.

Arthritis of the first metatarsophalangeal joint is known as **hallux rigidus**. It may occur along with hallux valgus and is important to recognise. Patients complain of a painful arc of movement, and OA changes will be seen on X-ray. A fusion of the first metatarsophangeal joint is considered if there is significant arthritis here.

Diabetic feet

Diabetic foot ulcers occur due to a combination of peripheral neuropathy resulting in unnoticed trauma, poor healing due to microvascular disease, and a susceptibility to infection caused by hyperglycaemia. Infections can be very difficult to control and osteomyelitis is common. Treatment is primary prevention with regular foot care, aggressive debridement of infected ulcers and offloading ulcerated areas with plaster casts. Amputation is performed in recalcitrant cases.

Charcot arthropathy is bone and joint destruction in the presence of peripheral neuropathy due to persistent loading of damaged joints combined with poor proprioception. The commonest cause is diabetes, but it is seen in other causes of neuropathy. First-line treatment is to cast the affected limb to allow bone healing to occur.

(26) Spine

Figure 26.1 Anatomy of the disc

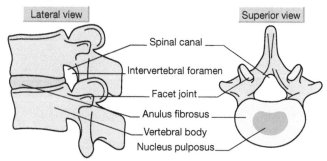

Lateral view   Superior view

Spinal canal
Intervertebral foramen
Facet joint
Anulus fibrosus
Vertebral body
Nucleus pulposus

Figure 26.3
T2 weighted sagittal MRI through the midline of the lumbar spine. The CSF is light. The cauda equina can be seen. The nucleus pulposus of the discs are dark because they are dehydrated, indicating that the discs are degenerate. There is a herniation of the L4–L5 disc which is causing significant narrowing of the spinal canal. Smaller disc herniations are seen at L3–L4 and L5–S1. In addition to the herniated discs, the facet joints are hypertrophic, indicating arthritis.This is exacerbating the narrowing of the canal caused by the disc prolapse and resulting in spinal stenosis

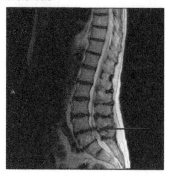

Figure 26.4 Clinical manifestations of root compression

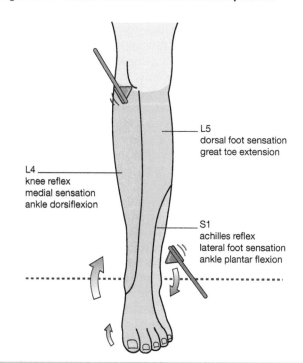

L5
dorsal foot sensation
great toe extension

L4
knee reflex
medial sensation
ankle dorsiflexion

S1
achilles reflex
lateral foot sensation
ankle plantar flexion

Figure 26.2 Normal MRI scans
(a) T1 weighted sagittal section through the midline of the lumbar spine. The discs appear grey, bones which contain fat are lighter. CSF is dark. Note that the intervertebral discs are of roughly equal height throughout

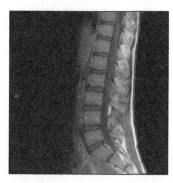

(b) T2 weighted sagittal MRI through the midline of the lumbar spine. CSF is bright because it consists mainly of water. The spinal cord and cauda equina can be seen clearly. The nucleus pulposus of the discs is bright because it contains large amounts of water. The annulus fibrosis is darker

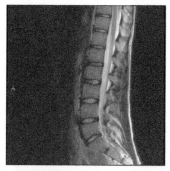

Figure 26.5 MRI of discitis

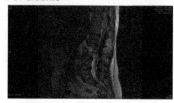

Figure 26.6 Red flag signs
Important features of the history which may indicate serious pathology are known as red flag signs. They include night pain, thoracic pain, fever, weight loss, age <20 or >55, neurological deficit, saddle anaesthesia or loss of bladder or bowel control and history of cancer

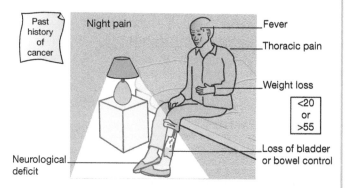

Past history of cancer

Night pain

Fever
Thoracic pain
Weight loss

<20 or >55

Loss of bladder or bowel control

Neurological deficit

Trauma and Orthopaedics at a Glance, First Edition. Henry Willmott.
© 2016 John Wiley & Sons, Ltd. Published 2016 by John Wiley & Sons, Ltd. Companion website: www.ataglanceseries.com/TandO

Back pain

Low back pain is very common in adults, affecting the majority of the population at some point in their lives. Most cases are self-limiting and do not need special investigations. Treatment consists of patient education, encouragement to stay mobile, physiotherapy and simple analgesia. NICE issued guidelines in 2009 that also suggested acupuncture and spinal manipulation may be effective.

There are some **diagnoses that must not be missed**:

- **infection** – discitis or epidural abscess;
- **fracture**;
- **malignancy** – primary or metastatic;
- **inflammatory conditions** – ankylosing spondylitis;
- **nerve root impingement** or **cauda equina syndrome**.

All patients should have a full history and examination, looking for red flag signs:

- thoracic pain;
- fever;
- unexpected weight loss;
- history of cancer;
- age of onset <20 years, >55 years;
- pain worse at night;
- neurological deficit – e.g. foot drop or paraesthesia;
- saddle anaesthesia or loss of bladder or bowel control.

Disc herniation

The vertebrae are separated by intervertebral discs, composed of two parts, made up like a car tyre. The outer layer is the tough fibrous **annulus fibrosus**. The centre section is a soft compressible **nucleus pulposus**.

As part of the natural ageing process, the nucleus pulposus becomes dehydrated and brittle. This is a common cause of mechanical back pain. The annulus fibrosus may also be affected and may split, allowing the nucleus pulposus to herniate out.

If a disc herniation compresses a nerve root, the result is shooting pain, numbness and weakness in the distribution of the affected nerve. This is known as **radiculopathy**. The commonest nerve roots to be affected are those supplying the sciatic nerve (L4-S3), causing sciatica. Typically sciatica pain radiates from the buttock as far as the sole of the foot.

The exact pattern of weakness, numbness and pain depends on which nerve root is affected:

Root	Sensation	Power	Reflex
L4	Medial foot and ankle	Ankle dorsiflexion	Patellar
L5	Dorsal foot, 1st webspace	Big toe extension	None
S1	Lateral foot and sole	Ankle plantarflexion	Ankle

The patient should be carefully examined for evidence of cauda equina syndrome (see below). If neurology is progressive or symptoms have been present for more than 6 weeks, an MRI should be organised. Most cases settle with conservative management as the herniated nucleus pulposus is resorbed and inflammation settles. Symptoms lasting more than 3 months are unlikely to resolve spontaneously and surgery to remove the herniated disc, a discectomy, may be considered

Cauda equina syndrome

The spinal cord terminates at L1. Below this level, the spinal canal is occupied by lower motor neurone nerves, collectively known as the cauda equina (horse's tail). The nerve roots are L2-S4 and supply most of the lower limb muscles and sensation of the perineum, including the bladder and rectal sphincters.

A large disc herniation can compress the nerves of the cauda equina. This is cauda equina syndrome and it is a surgical emergency.

Symptoms and signs include back pain, lower limb flaccid paralysis, loss of reflexes, paraesthesia of the perineum, loss of anal tone, faecal incontinence, painless retention of urine, overflow or stress incontinence of urine. Not all of these may be present.

Do a full neurological examination, which must be carefully documented. A rectal examination should be performed, assessing tone and sensation. If retention is suspected, catheterise and note the residual volume of urine in the bladder. Also note if the patient felt the catheter being inserted.

An **urgent MRI** will demonstrate herniation of a disc.

Treatment should be performed urgently and consists of surgical decompression of the spinal canal and evacuation of the herniated disc. Delaying surgery more than 24 hours significantly increases the risk of permanent nerve damage.

Spinal stenosis

In the elderly, a combination of disc degeneration and arthritis of the facet joints at the back of the spine can result in narrowing of the spinal canal, putting pressure on the spinal cord. The result is chronic pain in the legs, worse when walking and standing and relieved by leaning or sitting forwards. It resembles vascular claudication and may be differentiated by a normal vascular exam and careful history. Patients often notice that their exercise tolerance improves when walking around a supermarket – they are in fact opening up the spinal canal by leaning forward on the shopping trolley!

Treatment includes steroid epidural injection to reduce swelling, or surgical decompression of the canal (laminectomy).

Infections

A serious cause of back pain, **discitis** is infection within the intervertebral disc. The slow rate of blood flow within the disc allows bacteria from remote sources to become lodged and multiply. The result is severe back pain, fever and raised inflammatory markers. The elderly and immunosuppressed are most at risk. If left untreated an **epidural abscess** may form within the spinal canal and compress the spinal cord.

Investigations include inflammatory markers, blood cultures, MRI of the spine and a search for the source of bacteraemia, including cardiac echo to look for vegetations.

Treatment is a protracted course of antibiotics, often for several months. Presence of neurological symptoms may necessitate surgical decompression.

Tumours

Multiple myeloma is neoplasm of plasma cells and has a preference for the spine. Rarely, primary bone or neuronal primary tumours may occur in the spine or cord, but much more common is **metastasis** of cancer to the spine. **Breast, prostate, lung, thyroid and kidney** may all be responsible.

Patients may have weight loss, general malaise and pain worse at night, as well as symptoms of the primary tumour. A high index of suspicion is needed. **Investigations** include MRI, CT of the chest, abdomen and pelvis, urinary Bence Jones protein and tumour markers.

(27) Tumours

Figure 27.1   Sources of secondary bone lesion

In patients over 40 years of age, destructive bone lesions are most likely to be metastases from a primary tumour elsewhere. The commonest primary tumours are breast and prostate

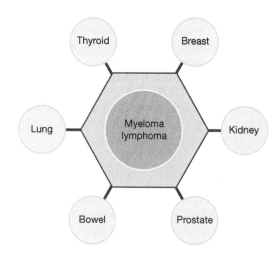

Figure 27.2   Identification of primary tumour site

- Take a thorough history and perform a full examination
- Obtain x-rays of the entire length of the affected bone and any other sites of pain, including the spine if indicated
- Blood tests should be taken
- CT of chest/abdomen/pelvis may reveal the primary tumour, lymphadenopathy or visceral metastases
- A bone scan will show any other bone deposits. 85% of primary tumours can be identified in this way

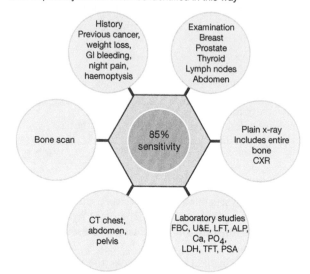

Figure 27.3   Bone scan

This bone scan demonstrates multiple bone lesions in a lady with metastatic breast cancer

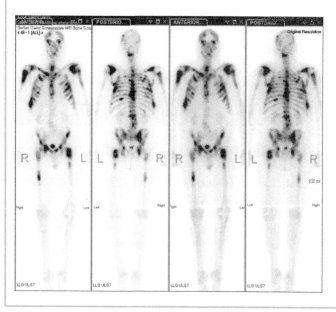

Figure 27.4   X-ray of bone lesion affecting right hemipelvis and femoral neck and pathological fracture of right neck of femur

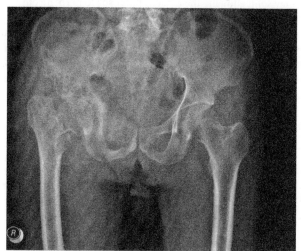

Metastatic bone tumours

The commonest tumour seen in bone is metastasis from a primary tumour elsewhere. Breast, prostate, lung, kidney, bowel and thyroid tumours all metastasise to bone. Older patients are usually affected.

Bone metastases may present with pain, which is classically worse at night, a pathological fracture that occurs in the absence of significant trauma, or as an incidental finding on an X-ray.

Management principles

Find the primary and stage the disease – in order to determine prognosis, the primary tumour must be sought. In some cases this may be known already, but if not, a full history and examination, CT chest-abdomen-pelvis, bone scan and tumour markers should be performed. Check serum calcium and liver function tests. X-ray the whole length of the affected bone to look for other lesions.

Determine the prognosis – close liaison with oncologists will determine the prognosis. In some cases radiotherapy or chemotherapy may be helpful, either to shrink the metastasis before surgery or as definitive treatment. Renal metastases respond to embolisation.

Determine fracture risk – if a fracture has not occurred, it is helpful to stratify the patient's risk of a fracture occurring. Mirels' score predicts risk of fracture:

Points	1	2	3
Appearance	Blastic	Mixed	Lytic
Size (diameter)	<1/3	1/3–2/3	>2/3
Site	Upper limb	Lower limb	Pertrochanteric
Pain	Mild	Moderate	Severe

Maximum score is 12. Score >8 correlates to a 33% risk of fracture and should be prophylactically fixed.

Stabilisation of the bone – generally speaking, intramedullary nailing is the preferred treatment. This allows the whole length of the bone to be supported, and the fixation will maintain strength even if the fracture does not heal. Reamings should be sent for histology to confirm the diagnosis. In some cases resection of the tumour may be indicated. This is generally the domain of specialist units.

Adjuvant therapy – after fixation the metastatic tumour will still need treatment. The oncologists may use radiotherapy or chemotherapy.

Primary bone tumours

Primary tumours of bone are rare. They tend to occur in younger patients. There are too many types of bone tumour to list here, but they may be broadly thought of as either benign or aggressive, and classified by the type of tissue they produce. When describing the appearance on an X-ray, you should consider:

- **Size** – describe in relation to the diameter of the normal bone – one-third, two-thirds, whole-diameter. Is it widening the bone or eroding it?
- **Location** – which bone, where in the bone (metaphysis, diaphysis, epiphysis), does it cross the growth plate, does it arise from the surface of the bone or from within the medullary cavity?
- **Zone of transition** – the boundary between the tumour and surrounding bone gives a clue as to the aggression of the tumour. Slow-growing benign tumours tend to have a very well-defined border, or narrow zone of transition. More aggressive tumours permeate into the surrounding bone, and as such are ill-defined with a wide zone of transition.
- **Matrix characteristics** – from what sort of material is the tumour made?
  - Osteosarcomas produce **bone** and can be seen on X-ray as thin wisps of bone extending out from the bone surface.
  - Chondrosarcomas and chondroblastomas produce **cartilage** and have a punched-out or lytic appearance on X-ray.
  - Fibroblastomas produce **collagen**, are often more benign and appear as bubbly lytic lesions on the X-ray.
  - Ewing's sarcoma is aggressive and rapidly produces **undifferentiated tissue**. Attempts to ossify the tissue result in an onion-skin appearance on X-ray.

Soft-tissue tumours

Tumours may arise from fat, muscle, blood vessels, nerves or synovium and may be benign or malignant. Tumours may metastasise, most commonly to the lungs, or exert pressure on adjacent neurovascular structures. Masses larger than 5 cm have a poor prognosis.

Staging

The principles of diagnostic work-up of bone or soft-tissue tumours are to obtain diagnosis, grade and stage. In almost all cases this is performed by a specialist tumour centre.

Imaging is performed in the form of plain X-ray of the whole bone, contrast-enhanced MRI, staging CT chest-abdomen-pelvis; also sometimes a bone scan to identify any other lesions.

Grading determines the aggression of the lesion and usually requires a **biopsy**. This may be performed as a needle aspiration, 'Tru-Cut' needle biopsy or open incisional biopsy. The biopsy tract will be contaminated with tumour cells and therefore will have to be included in any future resection. The biopsy should therefore only be performed in the specialist centre by the surgical team who will perform any future resection.

Staging determines size and location of the lesion. Broadly speaking, tumours can be confined to one muscular compartment, involve multiple compartments or have metastases.

Treatment

Treatment depends on the aggression and stage of the lesion.
- **Observation** – for benign asymptomatic lesions.
- **Aspiration or injection** – some bone cysts may be injected with steroid or bone marrow.
- **Curettage** –scraping out the lesion, often augmenting this with phenol or liquid nitrogen. The defect can be filled with bone graft.
- **Resection** – removal of part or all of the affected bone along with a margin of normal tissue. Reconstruction with endoprostheses can then be performed.
- **Chemotherapy and radiotherapy** – may be neoadjuvant (before surgery), adjuvant (after surgery) or as the definitive treatment.
- **Amputation** – indicated if the tumour cannot be safely resected with an adequate margin, the tumour involves major nerves or blood vessels, the tumour recurs after previous resection or the patient is not fit enough to undergo major reconstructive surgery.

(28) Rehabilitation

Figure 28.1 The multidisciplinary team

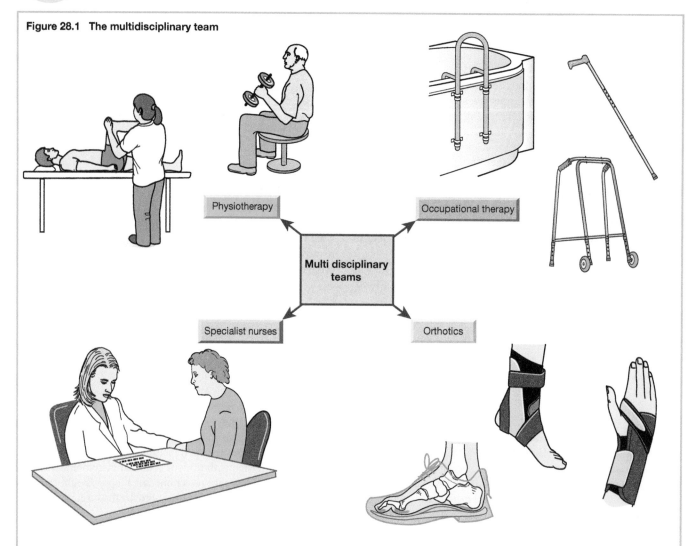

Figure 28.2 Prosthetic devices

(a) A simple body-powered pincer which is interchangeable with a selection of terminal devices designed for eating, (b) A powered ankle. A sensor in the forefoot detects when the patient is in the toe-off phase of gait. The motor behind the ankle creates plantar flexion to reproduce the action of the calf muscles and produce push-off, (c) A terminal device for running. The carbon fibre spring stores energy on landing, helping the athlete to cover greater distances with each stride., (d) A prosthesis for a patient with an above knee amputation. The knee joint is controlled by a microprocessor which locks and unlocks the joint at the appropriate phases of the gait cycle

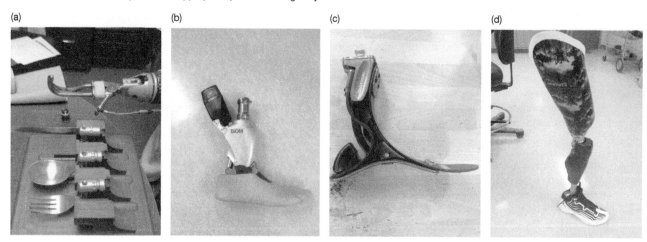

Trauma and Orthopaedics at a Glance, First Edition. Henry Willmott.
© 2016 John Wiley & Sons, Ltd. Published 2016 by John Wiley & Sons, Ltd. Companion website: www.ataglanceseries.com/TandO

Principles of rehabilitation

Rehabilitation of patients who have orthopaedic problems is one of the most important facets of the specialty. Without adequate therapy after injury, after surgery or in the presence of chronic disease, patients are unlikely to fulfil their functional potential. It is best achieved by a multidisciplinary team who liaise closely and work together.

Physiotherapy

Physiotherapy is a discipline concerned with the optimisation of physical function. Physiotherapists may be involved with the treatment of a range of orthopaedic, traumatic, surgical and medical problems. There are a variety of speciality areas within the profession, including sports, orthopaedic, geriatric, neurological, paediatric, cardiovascular, pulmonary and continence.

The techniques that are used most in orthopaedics include:
• Joint mobilisation and manipulation to restore range of movement after surgery or injury.
• Exercises to strengthen specific muscle groups to improve strength and movement in a coordinated manner.
• Neuromuscular and proprioceptive re-education to aid in preventing repeat injury or dislocation.
• Balance control and core stability to improve gait and posture and prevent falls.
• Interventional therapies for specific injuries including strapping, hot and cold packs and ultrasound therapy; prevention of further injury by guiding return to sport in a controlled manner.

Occupational therapy

Occupational therapy (OT) focuses on developing, maintaining and improving the patient's interaction with the environment in order to achieve tasks. The tasks may be simple activities of daily living such as feeding and washing, or much more complex such as using a computer or returning to work. There are three ways in which OTs work:
• adapting the environment
• modifying the task
• teaching new skills.

In orthopaedic practice this may mean providing sticks, frames, wheelchairs or hoists; providing higher chairs, grab handles, ramps or chairlifts in patients' homes; or liaising with employers or schools to help people with physical disabilities return to work.

OTs work closely with orthotists in the provision of aids and devices to achieve specific goals.

Orthotics

An orthotic is an externally applied device that modifies the structural and functional properties of the musculoskeletal system. They may act to:
• Correct malalignment: scoliosis of the spine and deformities of the knee or ankle can be braced with an orthotic.
• Limit movement: if a joint moves in an abnormal fashion, an orthotic can limit this. In cases such as spinal fractures, complete immobilisation or limitation of extreme movement is required.

• Support joints: wrist drop or foot drop may occur after nerve injury. Supporting the joint in a position of function allows the patient to use the hand to grip, or bear weight through the foot.
• Redistribute weight: if certain areas of the foot are overloaded this can generate pain. Insoles that reorientate the weightbearing axis and offload painful areas can alleviate this.

Orthotics can be custom made or supplied 'off the shelf' but in all cases an orthotist should be involved in the selection of the correct device and to ensure that it is properly fitted.

Prosthetics

Whereas an orthotic supports a limb, a prosthetic replaces a limb and has several components:
• Socket – transmits forces from the stump to the prosthesis.
• Means of suspension – keeps the socket securely attached to the stump. Types include suction sockets, suspension belts, neoprene or silicone sleeve.
• Joint mechanism – the knee is a difficult joint to reproduce as it must flex to allow foot clearance during the swing phase of gait, yet be locked solidly when weightbearing during the stance phase. There are a variety of different mechanisms, ranging from simple mechanical 'stance phase control' hinges, which lock in extension, to more complicated pneumatic, hydraulic or computer-controlled devices.
• Terminal device – the foot or hand. Feet can be simple solid ankles with a cushioned heel or much more complex energy-storing devices such as those worn by athletes. Hands may range from simple hooks, or pincers controlled by cables led from the shoulder, to complex myoelectric devices controlled by nerve impulses.

When an amputation is performed, the prosthetics service must be involved as soon as possible, ideally before the surgery if time allows. This enables the patient's demands to be assessed, aids with psychological adaptation and facilitates proper planning of the level of amputation and configuration of the stump.

Pre-hab and enhanced recovery

Recently a new concept called 'pre-habilitation' has been developed. This is a process of preparation for elective surgery whereby the issues that are usually tackled after surgery are addressed beforehand.

For example, a physiotherapist can meet a patient before an elective hip replacement to teach certain exercises to strengthen the muscles, retain range of movement and explain precautions to be taken to prevent dislocation. An occupational therapist can perform a home visit to arrange the provision of raised chairs, hand rails and advise alterations to the living space. Any medical issues such as diabetic control or hypertensive treatment can be optimised. On the day of surgery the patient is kept adequately hydrated. Anaesthetic techniques can be modified to ensure good postoperative analgesia without drowsiness or nausea.

Adopting these techniques shortens length of stay, reduces complications and improves patient satisfaction and outcome.

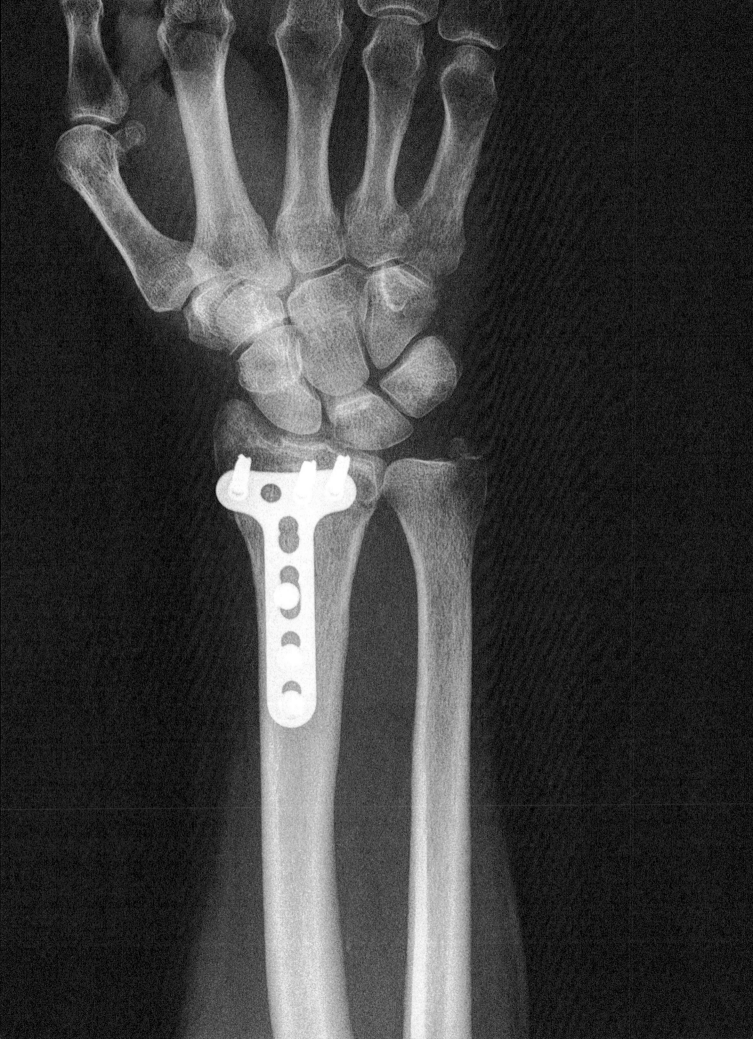

Paediatric orthopaedics

Part 3

Chapters

 Visit the companion website at **www.ataglanceseries.com/TandO** to test yourself on these topics.

29 Developmental dysplasia of hip (DDH)

Figure 29.1   Gluteal fold asymmetry

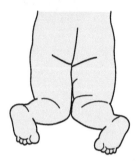

Figure 29.2   Limited abduction range

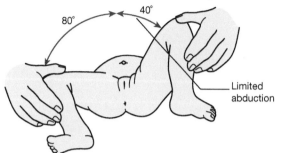

80° 40°

Limited abduction

Figure 29.3   Galeazzi test
Note difference in patella height

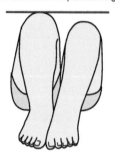

Figure 29.4   Barlow's test
Push femur backwards and feel for a clunk as the hip dislocates

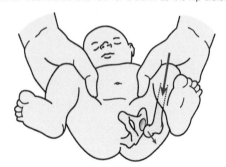

Figure 29.5   Ortolani's test
Abduct the hip and apply medial pressure with your index finger to reduce the hip back into joint with a palpable click

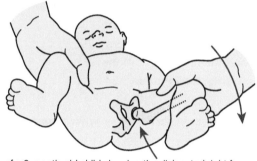

Figure 29.6 Ultrasound showing normal femoral head sitting inside acetabulum

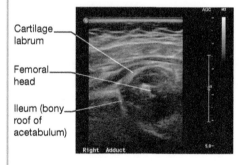

Cartilage labrum

Femoral head

Ileum (bony roof of acetabulum)

Figure 29.7 AP pelvis x-ray of a 9-month-old child showing the dislocated right femoral head above Hilgenreiner's line and lateral to Perkin's line. In contrast, the left femoral head is in the normal position

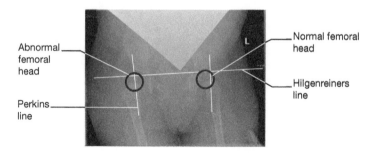

Abnormal femoral head

Perkins line

Normal femoral head

Hilgenreiners line

Figure 29.8 Treatment <6 months of age: Pavlik harness

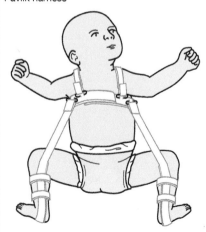

Figure 29.9 Treatment 6–24 months of age: EUA and hip spica

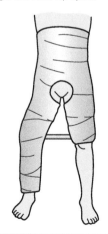

Figure 29.10 Treatment >24 months of age: open reduction and femoral or pelvic osteotomy

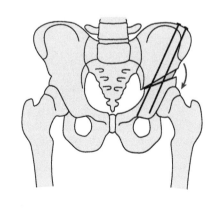

Trauma and Orthopaedics at a Glance, First Edition. Henry Willmott.
© 2016 John Wiley & Sons, Ltd. Published 2016 by John Wiley & Sons, Ltd. Companion website: www.ataglanceseries.com/TandO

Introduction

Developmental dysplasia of the hip (DDH) is a condition in which the femoral head does not lie congruently within the acetabulum. It is a spectrum of disease ranging from a femoral head that sits reduced for most of the time but can be pushed out of the acetabulum, often with a palpable or audible clunk (known as a 'clicking hip'), to a hip that is subluxed (partial contact remains between head and acetabulum), to the most severe form where the hip is dislocated and irreducible.

Failure to obtain a congruent reduction in a child means that the femoral head will not grow spherically and the acetabulum will not form properly. In later life this can lead to leg length discrepancy, abnormal gait, arthritis and pain.

Risk factors

Certain factors increase the risk of having DDH:
• breech position;
• first-born;
• oligohydramnios – these three factors restrict the space in the uterus for foetal development;
• female sex – higher levels of oestrogen result in increased ligamentous laxity;
• family history – 6% if normal parent; 12% if affected parent; 36% if affected sibling and parent.

DDH is commonest in the left hip because this is usually the side of the foetus that is pressed against the mother's spine. DDH is also associated with torticollis and metatarsus adductus. Collectively these conditions are known as packaging disorders, resulting from restricted intrauterine space.

Overall in the United Kingdom the risk of DDH is around 1:1000 live births. It is thought that up to 1 in 60 neonates may have a degree of DDH but the vast majority resolve spontaneously by 6 weeks. This limits the usefulness of neonatal screening tests.

Clinical signs

Always actively screen for the risk factors listed above.

Examination may reveal:
• **Gluteal fold asymmetry** – poor sensitivity but sometimes noted by healthcare workers or parents when changing nappies.
• **Abduction range** – a very simple test is to check the range of abduction of both hips. Asymmetry raises concerns.
• **Barlow's test** – detects a hip that can be dislocated posteriorly. Flex hip and knee to 90° and gently axially load, feeling for a clunk. Aide-memoire: *Barlow's push Backwards.*
• **Ortolani's test** – this test detects a hip that is already dislocated and can be reduced. Flex the hip and knee to 90° and keep your index finger on the greater trochanter. Abduct the hip gently and exert gentle forward pressure with your finger feeling for the hip popping back into joint. Aide memoire: *Ortolani's Open the legs.*
• **Galeazzi test** – flex hips and knees to 90° and look from the side for difference in patellar height indicating leg length discrepancy.

Imaging

The superior ossific nucleus of the femur, which will go on to form the femoral head, does not appear on X-rays until around 6 months of age. X-rays are therefore of limited use before this age.

Ultrasound – not only does US demonstrate the cartilaginous structures, it is dynamic, meaning that real-time screening can be performed as the hip is moved around. It also avoids exposure to radiation. The scans can be difficult to interpret (see Figure 29.6) but the key measurement is the angle between the bony roof of the acetabulum and the iliac wing. This is known as the α-angle. Normal value should be greater than 60°. An angle less than this indicates that the acetabulum is shallow and is unlikely to be able to keep the femoral head in joint.

X-ray – in children over 6 months of age the femoral head can be seen as a small dot. Two lines are drawn on the X-ray: Hilgenreiner's line across the triradiate cartilages of the acetabulae; Perkin's line perpendicular to Hilgenreiner's passing through the lateral edge of the roof of the acetabulum. The head should lie in the inferomedial quadrant formed by these two lines. Shenton's line can be traced and should be unbroken.

Arthrogram – if doubt remains as to whether the hip is transiently dislocating, subluxed or permanently dislocated, an arthrogram can be performed. Under anaesthetic, contrast is injected into the joint space and the hip screened under fluoroscopy in a variety of positions.

Treatment

Treatment is determined by age at presentation:

Under 6 months of age

A Pavlik harness is a device that holds the hip reduced. Straps keep the hip flexed and abducted. Too much flexion risks femoral nerve injury, too much abduction risks avascular necrosis of the femoral head. The harness should be worn for 23 hours per day. Reduction should be confirmed with US scans. The usual duration of treatment is 3 months.

6 months to 2 years

In this age bracket, all children should have an examination under anaesthetic (EUA) and arthrogram in order to determine if any structures are blocking concentric reduction.

If the hip is held reduced with the leg in a safe position (avoiding extremes of abduction or flexion), a hip spica cast can be applied for a total of 3 months.

If the hip is irreducible or only reduced in an extreme position, open reduction may be required. Most surgeons will defer this until the child is 18 months of age because the risks of surgery are less in older children.

Over 2 years of age

Children of this age need open reduction because the acetabulum will be full of fibrofatty tissue (pulvinar), the joint capsule will be stretched and baggy and there may be tendons interposed in the joint space. Surgery aims to remove obstacles to reduction and tighten up the capsule. Sometimes a femoral osteotomy is also required.

In children who present beyond 4 years of age, the acetabulum may be so shallow and poorly formed that a pelvic osteotomy must be performed to deepen and reorientate the acetabulum with the aim of improving coverage of the femoral head.

30 Other paediatric hip conditions

Figure 30.1 Perthes disease

(a) Presenting with a limp and pain in children between 4 and 8 years of age. The femoral head loses its blood supply and becomes flattened

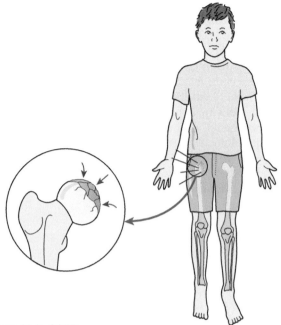

Figure 30.2 SCFE

(a) Presenting in an adolescent child and associated with obesity and endocrine abnormalities, symptoms may include limping and vague pain referred to the knee

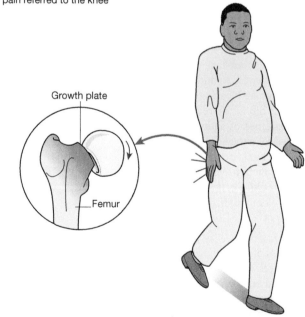

(b) X-ray of Perthes disease of the right femoral head in a six-year old. In the fragmentation stage, the epiphysis is smaller, and the physis irregular

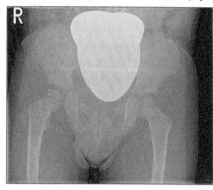

(c) X-ray of the same child as **Figure 30.1b**, 5 years later. The femoral head is flattened and widened but remains contained within the acetabulum. The risk of future osteoarthritis depends on the amount of remodelling which occurs

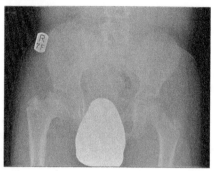

(b) Frog leg lateral x-ray of the pelvis showing the superior ossific nucleus of the right hip slipped backwards off the femoral neck. Klein's line does not intersect the femoral head

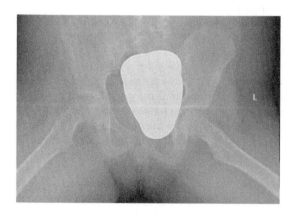

Perthes' disease

Perthes' disease is idiopathic osteonecrosis of the femoral head. As the head loses its blood supply it generates pain. As the dead bone collapses, the head loses its spherical shape.

Risk factors

Typically Caucasian boys aged 4–8 years are affected. The male:female ratio is 5:1. Risk factors are small stature, immature bone age and living in a poor urban environment with exposure to passive smoking.

Trauma and Orthopaedics at a Glance, First Edition. Henry Willmott.
© 2016 John Wiley & Sons, Ltd. Published 2016 by John Wiley & Sons, Ltd. Companion website: www.ataglanceseries.com/TandO

There is an association with thrombophilia and other clotting abnormalities implying that the disease is related to interruptions in the blood supply. Fifteen percent may be bilateral.

Symptoms

These are pain in the hip or groin. There is often an associated limp. Occasionally pain is referred to the knee.

Investigations

These should include an AP pelvis and frog-leg lateral X-ray of the hips (the child abducts and flexes the legs like a frog). The disease follows a chronological pattern, which can be seen on X-ray:

1 Initial stage –the X-ray may be normal. Occasionally a widened joint space may be seen, representing an effusion in the hip joint. As the disease progresses, sclerosis of the head may be seen.

2 Fragmentation– dead bone is resorbed resulting in subchondral fractures and the crescent sign. The extent of femoral head involvement can be evaluated at this stage and this reflects the prognosis – the more femoral head involved, the worse the prognosis.

3 Reossification – new bone is laid down. This process may take up to 18 months.

4 Remodelling – the head remodels until skeletal maturity. If it has remained well contained within the acetabulum, and the child was young at age of onset, it may remodel to a spherical shape, conveying a much better prognosis.

Prognosis

There are three main factors that determine the risk of arthritis and long-term pain.

- The **age** of the child: a younger child has more chance to remodel and will therefore do better. Children over 6 years old at onset have a poor prognosis.
- The **extent** of femoral head involvement: if more of the femoral head is involved, the outcome is worse. The lateral one-third of the femoral head is the main weightbearing section. If this has significantly collapsed, arthritis may result.
- **Abduction contracture**: if the hip loses significant abduction, remodelling will be limited and the outcome less favourable.

Treatment

Most cases are treated conservatively with activity modification and periods of partial weightbearing when the hip is painful. In the past braces and traction were used but these have not been shown to improve long-term results.

The child should be carefully monitored for loss of abduction and decreased range of movement as this may indicate that the head is no longer contained within the acetabulum. X-rays should be performed periodically. If the head is no longer contained within the cup, surgery is indicated. This may be a femoral osteotomy, a pelvic osteotomy or a combination of both.

Slipped capital femoral epiphysis

Slipped capital femoral epiphysis (SCFE, formerly known as slipped upper femoral epiphysis – SUFE), is caused by a weakness in the growth plate of the femoral head resulting in the femoral neck slipping on the femoral head.

Classification

Chronicity

- Acute (symptoms for less than 3 weeks).
- Chronic (symptoms for more than 3 weeks).
- Acute on chronic (background pain with sudden exacerbation).

Stability

The slip may be thought of as stable if the child is able to weight-bear, with or without crutches. If the child cannot bear weight it is unstable. Unstable slips have approximately a 50% risk of going on to develop the catastrophic complication of avascular necrosis, whereas stable slips almost never have this problem.

Risk factors

These include:
- age 10–16 years;
- male sex;
- obesity;
- Afro-Caribbean origin;
- endocrinopathy including hypothyroidism and hypogonadism;
- positive family history.

Twenty-five percent may be bilateral.

Symptoms and signs

The child often presents with a limp and groin pain. The pain is frequently referred to the knee. Any child in this age group with unexplained knee pain should have X-rays of their hips.

Investigations

X-rays are the mainstay. AP pelvis and frog-leg lateral should be obtained. The frog-leg view is the most sensitive. Trace the superior border of the femoral neck and extrapolate it beyond the growth plate. This line, known as Klein's line, should intersect the lateral third of the femoral head. In SCFE, the head slips below Klein's line.

Treatment

For most cases, the aim of surgery is to prevent the slip from progressing any further. This is achieved by 'pinning in situ'. A single screw is passed across the growth plate to anchor it in position. In very severe slips, an open reduction and internal fixation may be considered. This is challenging surgery and exposes the head to the risk of avascular necrosis.

If the child is very high risk for a slip on the other side, prophylactic pinning may be considered. Indications for this would be a child under 10 years, or with a known endocrinopathy.

Septic arthritis and transient synovitis

Septic arthritis of the hip is covered in Chapter 7. A cause of hip pain that often mimics septic arthritis is transient synovitis or 'irritable hip'. The exact aetiology is unknown, but the typical history is of a child of 2–5 years of age with a sudden-onset limp and complaint of hip pain. It may be associated with gastroenteritis or viral upper respiratory tract infection (URTI). The hip develops an effusion and the child holds the hip flexed and externally rotated, and is unwilling to move it.

Blood tests reveal normal or mildly elevated inflammatory markers and a normal white cell count. The child is usually afebrile.

Transient synovitis is self-limiting and usually responds quickly to NSAIDs.

Septic arthritis, on the other hand, is very serious. Kocher developed a set of diagnostic criteria to differentiate a septic joint from an irritable joint:
- WBC >12,000 cells/μL;
- inability to bear weight;
- fever >38.5°C;
- erythrocyte sedimentation rate (ESR) >40 mm/h.

Four positive criteria have a 99% predictive value for septic arthritis, three criteria 93%, two criteria 40% and one criterion 3%. If in doubt, an ultrasound-guided aspiration of the hip will confirm the diagnosis.

31 Paediatric spinal disorders

Figure 31.1 Clinical signs of scoliosis
(a) Shoulder slope and scapular prominence
(b) Adam's forward bent test eliminates lumbar compensation

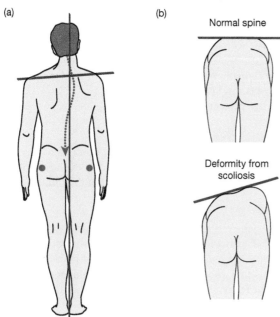

Figure 31.2 Measurement of curve magnitude
Identify the apex. Then identify the two end vertebrae. These are the most tilted vertebrae either side of the apex. The Cobb angle is the angle between the two end vertebrae and is a measurement of the severity of the curve

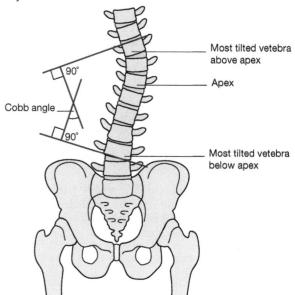

Figure 31.3 Congenital scoliosis
Each growing vertebra has two growth centres. Failure of adjacent vertebrae to separate or failure of half a vertebra to grow leads to rapidly progressive scoliosis in an infant

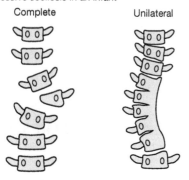

Figure 31.5 Spina bifida
Failure of the posterior elements of the spinal canal to close results in exposure of the neural elements in the midline

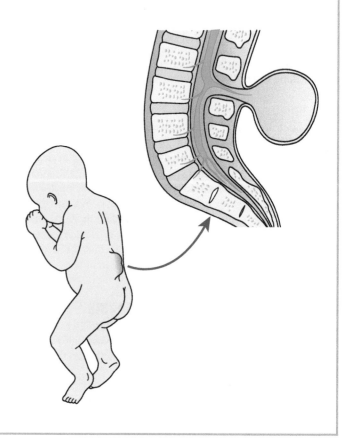

Figure 31.4 Spondylolysis
A stress fracture in the pars interarticularis may occur after repeated hyperextension exercises. This is painful. Severe cases result in forward slippage of the vertebra, know as spondylolisthesis. This may trap nerve roots and cause symptoms in the lower limbs

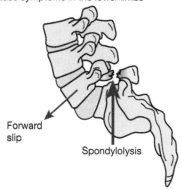

Trauma and Orthopaedics at a Glance, First Edition. Henry Willmott.
© 2016 John Wiley & Sons, Ltd. Published 2016 by John Wiley & Sons, Ltd. Companion website: www.ataglanceseries.com/TandO

Scoliosis

Scoliosis is a deformity of the spine in three planes – rotation, lateral bending and lordosis. In mild cases it may be barely noticeable. In moderate cases prominence of the ribs on one side produces cosmetic concerns. In severe cases pulmonary insufficiency results from restriction of thoracic expansion.

Scoliosis can be classified into several groups.

Idiopathic scoliosis

This is the commonest type of scoliosis. It may occur as an infant (<3 years), a juvenile (3–10 years) or an adolescent (>10 years). The curve may be single (lumbar or thoracic), or double involving both lumbar and thoracic segments. The commonest subtype is adolescent idiopathic scoliosis with a right thoracic curve.

Diagnosis and screening

The child or a parent may notice one shoulder blade is more prominent than the other, or the shoulders or hips appear at different levels. The child may compensate very effectively for a thoracic curve by bending the lumbar spine to stay upright. In order to eliminate this compensation, perform the **Adams' forward bend test**: ask the child to bend at the waist and look from behind at the level of the scapulae. The alternative is to sit the child down with the hips bent to 90°. This eliminates lumbar compensation.

Idiopathic scoliosis is not painful and does not cause neurological symptoms. Presence of pain or neurological symptoms should raise concerns of more serious pathology.

X-rays are the first investigation. The whole spine should be imaged on one PA film.

Measurement of curve magnitude

Draw a plumb line from the middle of C7 to the middle of the sacrum. This represents the midline. Try to identify where the curve starts and ends: the disc spaces will be open on one side and closed on the other. The point at which the disc orientation changes is the end vertebra. Next measure the Cobb angle between the two end vertebrae. This parameter defines the magnitude of the curve.

Risk of progression

Some curves will not progress, and can therefore be treated conservatively. Others will progress rapidly and may need treatment with a brace or surgery. There are several risk factors that predict progression. The most important risk factors are:

- female sex
- young age
- premenarche
- skeletal immaturity
- Cobb angle >50°
- progression >5° over two serial X-rays.

Treatment

As a rule of thumb the treatment of idiopathic scoliosis is determined by the Cobb angle; treatment should be:

- **<25° – observe**
- **25–40° – brace**
- **>40° – consider surgery especially if prepubertal.**

Congenital scoliosis

Failure of adjacent vertebrae to separate, or failure of half a vertebra to grow, results in a mismatch between left and right halves of the spine. The result is a rapidly progressive scoliosis in an infant.

Congenital scoliosis is often associated with other congenital abnormalities such as cardiac, renal, genitourinary and facial abnormalities. In addition, restriction of thoracic capacity at an early age limits development of the lungs.

Surgery is difficult and dangerous with risk of neurological injury and short stature as an adult.

Neuromuscular scoliosis

Conditions that alter the normal tone of muscles can result in scoliosis in the growing child. Underlying conditions may be paralytic (e.g. polio), muscle weakness (e.g. muscular dystrophy) or upper motor neurone (e.g. cerebral palsy). The curves tend to be long and C-shaped involving both lumbar and thoracic segments. Treatment may include bracing, adapting wheelchair cushions to allow sitting, or surgical correction.

Spondylolysis

This is a defect in the pars interarticularis – the section of bone between the superior and inferior parts of the facet joint. There are a number of reasons why the defect may be present in adults, but in adolescents the commonest reason is a stress fracture due to repeated hyperextension. Sportsmen and gymnasts are typically affected, complaining of low back pain.

X-rays may show the fracture, although it can be difficult to see. Oblique X-rays may help. Better is a CT or SPECT scan (a technique that combines a bone scan with a CT).

Mild cases settle spontaneously with activity modification. More severe cases, where the fracture has displaced, may result in spondylolisthesis – forward slippage of a lumbar vertebra over another. If this occurs, reduction and fixation may be required.

Spina bifida

Failure of the foetal neural tube to close properly results in exposure of the spinal cord posteriorly. There are varying degrees of severity, ranging from an occult spina bifida manifest as a small hairy patch on the back, to a myelomeningocoele, where the dura is exposed to the environment. The aetiology is multifactorial but includes maternal folate deficiency during pregnancy.

Orthopaedic manifestations of spina bifida are varied but include scoliosis, hip dysplasia, knee deformities, and foot and ankle contractures and deformities. The level of spinal involvement determines the independence and level of function of the individual.

32 Paediatric foot conditions

Figure 32.1 Congenital talipes equinovarus–the foot is rigid
This condition may be associated with DDH, torticollis, arthrogryposis
(multiple joint contractures) and spina bifida

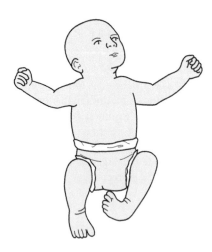

Figure 32.2 Denis-Browne boots
After serial casting following the Ponseti method, the child is put into
this splint, which is worn full time for three months and then at night
and nap time for three years

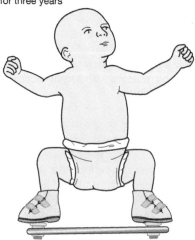

Figure 32.3 Tarsal coalition is abnormal connections between
bones of the foot resulting in rigid flat foot deformity:
(a) The 'anteater' sign: a bony connection between the calcaneum
and the navicular

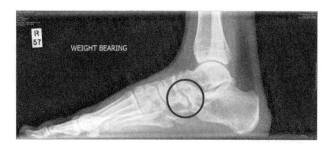

WEIGHT BEARING

(b) The 'C' sign: A bony connection between the talus and the
calcaneum

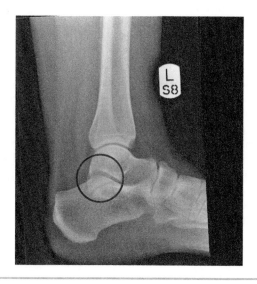

Trauma and Orthopaedics at a Glance, First Edition. Henry Willmott.
© 2016 John Wiley & Sons, Ltd. Published 2016 by John Wiley & Sons, Ltd. Companion website: www.ataglanceseries.com/TandO

Congenital talipes equinovarus (CTEV)

Also known as 'club foot', CTEV has an incidence in the UK of around 2/1000, with three-quarters of cases occurring in males. Twenty-five percent of cases have a positive family history and 50% of cases are bilateral.

A number of aetiological theories exist, including abnormalities in muscles or nerves and intrauterine moulding. It is associated with 'packaging deformities', including developmental dysplasia of the hip (DDH) and torticollis, which occur when intrauterine space is restricted due to twins or oligohydramnios. CTEV may also be associated with arthrogryposis (multiple joint contractures), spina bifida or other syndromes.

The deformity affects the foot and calf. The foot has four deformities (an aide-memoire is the acronym **CAVE**):
- **Cavus** – a high arch and plantar-flexed first ray.
- **Adductus** of the midfoot – the foot turns inwards.
- **Varus** of the hindfoot – together this comprises supination.
- **Equinus** – a tight Achilles tendon.

In addition to these deformities, the calf muscles are hypotrophic and the foot is smaller, requiring different shoe sizes in later life.

Treatment

Ponseti technique
The deformity can be gradually corrected over several weeks with serial casts. The treatment regimen is started immediately from birth. Moulded plaster casts are applied at weekly intervals for around 3 months.

The foot deformities are corrected sequentially, starting with correction of cavus by raising the first ray. Then the hindfoot adductus and varus are corrected simultaneously. Finally, the equinus deformity is addressed by applying dorsiflexion at the ankle. In most hospitals, the casts are applied by specialist physiotherapists.

Around 90% of cases have a very tight Achilles tendon, which prevents correction of the equinus. The tendon is therefore released surgically. This minor procedure can be done under local anaesthetic in clinic. A small blade is inserted through a tiny incision to divide the tendon beneath the skin.

Once the foot is in an acceptable position, it is put into a final cast for 3 weeks. Once this cast is removed, there is a natural tendency for recurrence, so the foot must be held corrected for some time. This is achieved with 'Denis Browne boots'. Two soft boots connected by a bar hold the feet adducted at shoulder width. The child wears the boots full-time for 3 months, and then at night-time and nap-time for 3 years. Although this sounds like an ordeal, most children and their parents manage well.

Recurrent deformity after Ponseti casting
The commonest reason for recurrence is poor compliance with the Denis Browne boots. Mild recurrence may respond to another few weeks of casting.

Resistant CTEV
Failure to respond to Ponseti casting is known as resistant CTEV. This is commoner in syndromic conditions such as arthrogryposis. In these cases, surgical correction may be required. Tight ligaments are divided, tendons lengthened and the bones aligned and held with wires. Risk of wound breakdown, neurovascular injury, growth arrest and overcorrection exist.

Tarsal coalition

The tarsal bones comprise the talus, navicular, cuboid and three cuneiforms. Movement between them maintains a flexible arch and is important for normal function of the midfoot. Failure of the bones to separate during development results in abnormal rigid connections between the tarsal bones. This is known as tarsal coalition.

The incidence is around 1%, with a male to female ratio of around 2:1. There are two main types of coalition, which account for 90% of cases: calcaneonavicular coalition (CNC) and talocalcaneal coalition (TCC), although coalitions may occur between any of the tarsal bones.

	Proportion of cases	Bilaterality	Age of presentation
CNC	40%	30%	8–12 years
TCC	50%	50%	12–16 years
TNC	8%	5%	Variable
Other	2%		

CNC: calcaneonavicular; TCC: talocalcaneal; TNC: talonavicular.

Symptoms and signs
Although the coalition will be present from birth, it is flexible cartilage until ossification begins. Coalitions therefore do not present until around the second decade (earlier for CNC). The child may complain of frequent ankle sprains or pain following sports. Pain may be medial or lateral. As the condition progresses, restricted movement may be noted and progressive flattening of the foot will develop.

Investigation
Imaging should initially be in the form of plain X-rays. In CNC, oblique images of the foot may show an osseous bar between the calcaneum and the navicular. This is known as the anteater sign as it is said to resemble the nose of an aardvark. In TCC, irregularity of the posterior facet of the calcaneum may be seen on the lateral view, along with the 'C-sign'.

CT or MRI is the next step. The latter is perhaps more useful because it shows the full extent of a fibrous coalition as well as the presence of any other coalitions.

Treatment
In the first instance the foot should be rested for 6 weeks in a below-knee cast or fixed-angle walker boot. In mild cases this resolves the pain and with activity modification no further treatment is required.

If this fails to settle symptoms, or restriction of sporting activity is unacceptable to the patient, resection of the coalition can be performed. This may be open or arthroscopic. Recurrence is frequent and the surgeon may try interposing fat or muscle between the bones to prevent this. In recurrent cases, or if the majority of the joint surface is involved, subtalar fusion can be performed. Although this will not restore movement, the aim is to achieve a painless fusion in a position which maintains the arch.

Idiopathic flat foot

This is very common, especially in Afro-Caribbean people. The arch usually restores when standing on tiptoes or when the big toe is pushed into dorsiflexion (Jack's test). Pain or rigidity should prompt investigation for coalition. Insoles and orthotics do not improve function and are not recommended. Reassurance is normally all that is needed.

33 Neuromuscular conditions

Figure 33.1 Classification of cerebral palsy

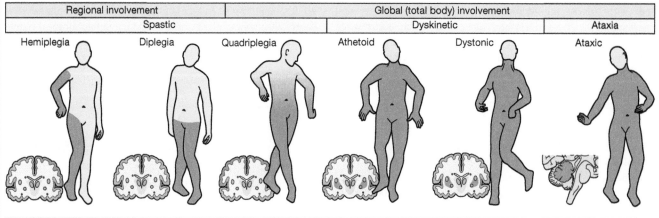

Regional involvement			Global (total body) involvement		
Spastic			Dyskinetic		Ataxia
Hemiplegia	Diplegia	Quadriplegia	Athetoid	Dystonic	Ataxic

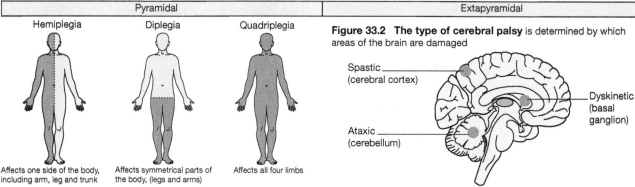

Pyramidal			Extapyramidal
Hemiplegia	Diplegia	Quadriplegia	

Affects one side of the body, including arm, leg and trunk

Affects symmetrical parts of the body, (legs and arms)

Affects all four limbs

Figure 33.2 The type of cerebral palsy is determined by which areas of the brain are damaged

Spastic (cerebral cortex)

Dyskinetic (basal ganglion)

Ataxic (cerebellum)

Figure 33.3 Gait abnormalities in spastic cerebral palsy

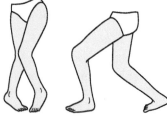
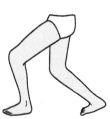
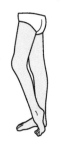
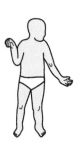
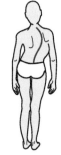

1. Scissor gait **2.** Crouch gait **3.** Toe-walking gait **4.** Upper limb posturing **5.** Scoliosis

Figure 33.4 Orthotic options for cerebral palsy

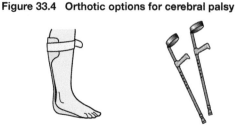

(a) Ankle-foot-orthosis (AFO)

(b) Crutches

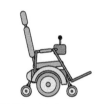

(c) Wheeled walker frame

(d) Wheelchair

Figure 33.5 Gower's sign In muscular dystrophy, the child has proximal leg weakness. When sitting on the floor, they are unable to rise to a standing position directly. Instead, they use their hands to 'climb up' their own legs

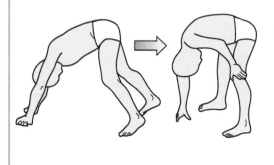

Figure 33.6 Cavovarus foot, typical of HMSN (Charcot-Marie-tooth disease)
Muscle imbalance results in a high arch (cavus) and hindfoot varus. There is often muscle wasting, a waddling gait and clawing of the toes. This deformity may also be caused by spinal pathologies, so always examine for this

Varus

High arch (cavus)

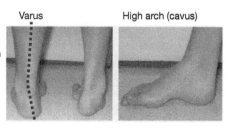

Trauma and Orthopaedics at a Glance, First Edition. Henry Willmott.
© 2016 John Wiley & Sons, Ltd. Published 2016 by John Wiley & Sons, Ltd. Companion website: www.ataglanceseries.com/TandO

Cerebral palsy (CP)

Cerebral palsy is a non-progressive neuromuscular disorder with age of onset before 2 years, due to injury to the immature brain. It is important to appreciate that although the neurological condition is non-progressive, the musculoskeletal manifestations may progress in the form of soft-tissue contractures, joint subluxation and growth disturbance

The **aetiology** is often unknown but may include:
- prenatal infection (toxoplasmosis, rubella, CMV, herpes simplex);
- intrauterine oxygen deficiency;
- prematurity;
- anoxic brain injury;
- meningitis.

Classification

CP is classified by physiology and anatomy.

Anatomy (how much of the body is affected?):
- Hemiplegic – one arm and one leg affected.
- Diplegic – both arms or both legs.
- Total involvement – all four limbs plus spinal muscles.

Physiology (how are the muscles affected?):
- Spastic – increased muscle tone. This is the commonest type.
- Ataxic – cerebellar involvement affecting fine motor control.
- Dyskinetic/athetoid – abnormal tone often associated with involuntary movements.
- Mixed.

Clinical manifestations

As an upper motor neurone disorder, CP causes mixed spasticity and weakness. This results in imbalanced pull of muscles across joints. Joint contractures may occur. Initially these are correctible with manipulation but with time they become fixed. The persistent abnormal pull of muscles affects the growth of bones, which become deformed. Joints may eventually subluxate or dislocate. Secondary manifestations may include seizures, learning difficulty, apraxia and dysarthria.

Treatment

There are a variety of treatment modalities:
- Physiotherapy: manipulation to prevent contractures from developing.
- Drugs: muscle relaxants such as baclofen (GABA agonist) reduce spasticity. Botox (botulinum toxin) acts to block acetylcholine action at the neuromuscular junction.
- Orthotics: splints and braces treat and prevent deformity and improve gait.
- Occupational and speech therapy: to optimise function.
- Surgery: release of tight soft tissues and tendons; osteotomies to correct deformed bones; selective cutting of dorsal nerve roots as they leave the spinal cord (rhizotomy); correction of spinal scoliosis if a child is unable to sit upright.

Arthrogryposis

Derived from the Greek for 'curved joints', arthrogryposis multiplex congenita is a rare congenital condition causing multiple stiff joints. There are many subtypes, not all of which are fully understood. The aetiology is often unknown but may be due to abnormal muscle (myopathic), abnormal nerves or reduced numbers of anterior horn cells (neuropathic), or mixed factors.

Individuals may be variably affected but classically, shoulders are internally rotated, elbows extended, wrists and fingers flexed, hips flexed and externally rotated and sometimes dislocated, knees flexed and feet clubbed. There are no skin creases over the joints. Intelligence is usually normal.

Treatment is with passive manipulation and serial casting. Older children may require soft-tissue releases or corrective osteotomies to allow elbow flexion so they can feed themselves. Hip dislocation and club-foot correction are difficult and recurrence is common.

Myopathies

There are many conditions affecting muscle function. Some of the more common are listed below:
- **Duchenne's muscular dystrophy** – X-linked recessive condition caused by lack of a muscle protein called dystrophin. The result is progressive weakness of muscles. Signs include clumsy walking, lumbar lordosis, calf pseudohypertrophy due to fatty infiltration, and Gowers' sign (calf weakness causing inability to get off the floor without using the arms). Children lose ambulation at an average age of 10 years and die from respiratory failure at 20.
- **Becker's dystrophy** – less severe form of Duchenne's where some functioning dystrophin remains. Occurs exclusively in red-green colour-blind boys.
- **Fascioscapulohumeral dystrophy** – autosomal dominant condition, presenting at around 6–20 years old, which affects the muscles of the upper limb and face causing winging of the scapulae and facial abnormalities.

Hereditary motor sensory neuropathy (HMSN)

Formerly known as Charcot–Marie–Tooth disease, this condition affects nerve conduction, resulting in mixed sensory and motor deficits.

There are two main subtypes. **Type 1** is due to demyelination of nerves and is inherited in an autosomal dominant pattern, whereas **type 2** is due to direct axonal death and is autosomal recessive. Further subtypes exist but are much rarer.

Motor function of the hands and feet is affected, specifically weakness of intrinsic muscles, peroneus brevis and tibialis anterior. The result is a cavovarus (high arch and inverted) foot with clawing of the toes along with wasting and clawing in the hands.

Treatment is surgical in the form of osteotomies to correct the foot deformity along with tendon transfers to improve eversion and extension at the ankle.

Friedreich's ataxia

A rare autosomal recessive condition caused by an absent mitochondrial iron-binding protein called frataxin, resulting in damage to nerves and dorsal root ganglia.

Patients present in their 20s with a wide-based gait, high-arched foot, scoliosis and cardiomyopathy. Examination reveals ataxia, areflexia and nystagmus. Affected individuals are usually wheelchair bound by age 30 and die from cardiomyopathy around 50.

34 Lower limb alignment

Figure 34.1   Staheli rotational profile

(a) Forefoot progression angle: Observe the child walking to give an overall impression of in-or-out-toeing

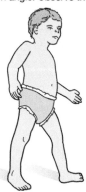
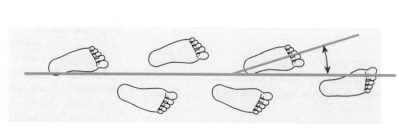

(b) Hip internal rotation. With the child in the prone position, examine from the end of the couch, comparing both sides

(c) Hip external rotation. Stabilise the pelvis with your hand to prevent pelvic tilt

(e) Heel bisector line: First find the transmalleolar line which connects the medial and lateral malleoli. A line perpendicular to this normally passes through 2nd/3rd webspace. Curvature of the lateral border of the foot represents metatarsus adductus

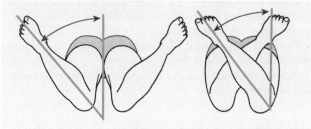

(d) Thigh foot angle. Examine from above and estimate the angle subtended by the long axis of the foot and the femur

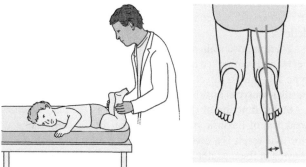

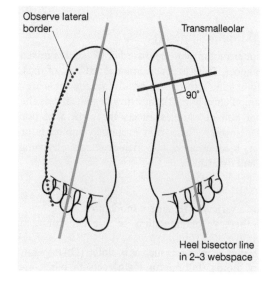

Observe lateral border

Transmalleolar

90°

Heel bisector line in 2–3 webspace

Figure 34.2   Natural variation of tibiofemoral angle with age

When assessing a child with varus or valgus knees, it is important to appreciate the natural progression from varus at birth, to neutral at age 2, to valgus in adulthood. 'Normal' is two standard diviations either side of the mean

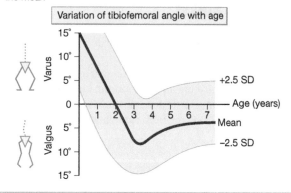

Variation of tibiofemoral angle with age

Varus   15°
10°
5°
0° — Age (years) — +2.5 SD
5°   Mean
Valgus 10°   –2.5 SD
15°
1 2 3 4 5 6 7

Figure 34.3   X-ray of rickets

Note the widened physes, flared metaphyses and bowing of the tibiae

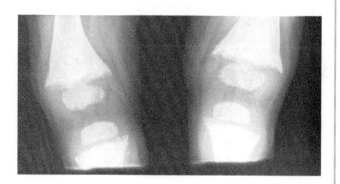

Trauma and Orthopaedics at a Glance, First Edition. Henry Willmott.
© 2016 John Wiley & Sons, Ltd. Published 2016 by John Wiley & Sons, Ltd. Companion website: www.ataglanceseries.com/TandO

Rotational alignment

A common parental concern that prompts attendance at a paediatric orthopaedic clinic is a child who walks 'pigeon-toed', or with feet turned inwards, properly known as *in-toeing gait*.

Natural progression

Rotational alignment is measured by the foot progression angle, which is the angle of the long axis of the foot with respect to the sagittal plane. Neonates naturally have a negative foot progression angle (in-toeing), whereas adults naturally have a positive foot progression angle (out-toeing). Progression from in-toeing to out-toeing happens over several years and as with all such processes, there is a range of normality. Some children may become out-toeing more quickly, some more slowly.

The rotational transition from in- to out-toeing occurs at three sites:

Femoral neck – if a femur is viewed from above, the neck is seen to be at an angle to the femoral condyles. This is known as femoral anteversion. At birth the normal value is 30–40°, whereas in adulthood the normal value is 15°. Children therefore have increased femoral anteversion, which decreases with time.

Tibial shaft – along the length of the tibia there is a twist. This is measured by the difference between the axis of the knee proximally and the axis of the two malleoli distally. Children have internal tibial torsion, which decreases with time.

Foot – the long axis of the foot also changes with maturity. A neonate's foot is shaped rather like a coffee bean – the lateral border is curved whereas an adult has a straight lateral border. This is known as metatarsus adductus. It is measured by the heel bisector angle, which in neonates passes through the fourth toe, in adults the second toe.

Causes of in-toeing gait

In-toeing is due to internal rotation of the limb. Determining the site of rotation is achieved by performing an examination known as the *Staheli rotational profile* (see illustration). There are three sites at which the deformity may arise:

- **Increased femoral anteversion** – hip internal rotation >70° and external rotation <20°.
- **Increased tibial torsion** – thigh–foot angle is less than −10°.
- **Metatarsus adductus** – the heel-bisector line passes lateral to the third toe.

Most cases presenting to the clinic are within the normal range; the parents and child can be reassured.

Pathological in-toeing

The presence of these features should arouse suspicion for a pathological cause:

- asymmetry
- pain
- spasticity
- progression in the wrong direction
- marked deviation from normal values.

  Potential causes for pathological in-toeing include:
- cerebral palsy
- spina bifida
- arthrogryposis
- developmental dysplasia of the hip (DDH)
- Perthes' disease

- slipped capital femoral epiphysis (SCFE)
- post-traumatic/growth disturbance.

Treatment is discussed in the relevant chapters.

Coronal alignment (varus/valgus)

Just as with rotational alignment, the lower limbs change their coronal alignment with maturity. Neonates are naturally bow-legged (varus), whereas adults are slightly knock-kneed (valgus).

Average alignment varies with age:

- Birth: 15° varus
- 2 years: neutral
- 3 years: 10° valgus
- 5 years through to adulthood: 6° valgus.

'Normality' is two-standard deviations (roughly 15°) either side of these values, as illustrated in Figure 34.2. Most cases seen in the clinic fall into this normal range and need nothing more than reassurance and monitoring.

Pathological varus/valgus

The features suggestive of a pathological process are:

- asymmetry;
- pain;
- progression in the wrong direction;
- alignment grossly outside the normal range;
- other generalised skeletal abnormalities.

  Potential causes include:

- **Rickets** – defective mineralisation of the growth plate results in varus (bowing) at the knees. X-rays show widened metaphyses, cupping of the physis and curved bones. Causes include lack of sunlight, particularly in black or Asian children living in northern latitudes; lack of dietary calcium or vitamin D; congenital absence of liver enzymes to hydroxylate vitamin D to its active form; congenital absence of vitamin D receptors; and renal phosphate loss. Treatment is to find the underlying cause and treat with dietary supplements.
- **Blount's disease** – an inherited condition that uniquely affects black children, Blount's disease is premature closure of the posteromedial part of the proximal tibial growth plate. The result is progressive varus deformity and internal rotation of the tibia at the knee. It is associated with obesity and it is postulated that increased loads across the growth plate may be a contributory factor. Treatment may include corrective osteotomy or correction with an external fixator frame.
- **Growth disturbance** – trauma or infection can damage the growth plate of tibia or femur. Ask specifically for this in the history. X-rays may show a malunited fracture or a bony bar crossing the growth plate and tethering one side. Treatment options include corrective osteotomy, resection of a bony bar or selective closure of the contralateral side of the growth plate with a staple.
- **Skeletal dysplasias** – there are many conditions that affect generalised growth of the skeleton. Each has its own radiographic and clinical characteristics, but the clue is that multiple sites including the upper limbs and spine may be involved.
- **Tibial bowing** – although strictly speaking not a cause of coronal plane deformity at the knee, tibial bowing has a similar appearance at first glance. However, careful examination reveals deformity within the tibial shaft rather than the knee joint. There are several causes, including neurofibromatosis, failure of tibial development (tibial hemimelia), failure of fibular development (fibular hemimelia) or a simple packaging deformity due to lack of intrauterine space. Treatment is dependent upon the cause.

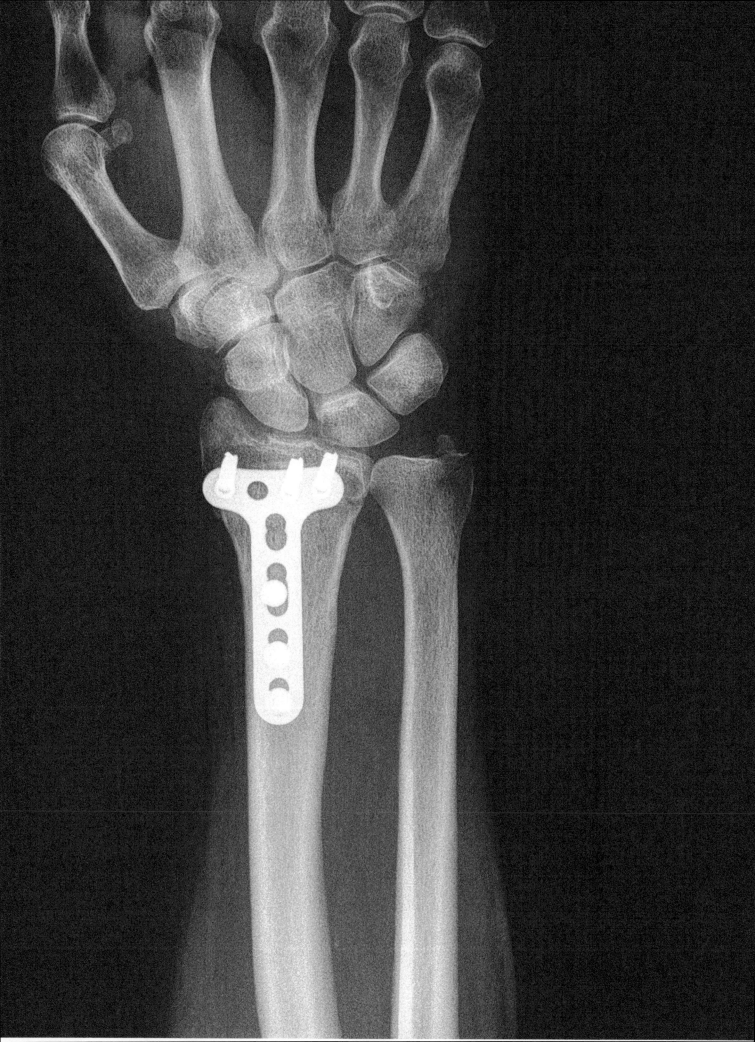

Trauma

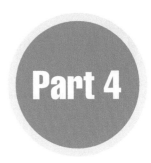

Part 4

Chapters

 Visit the companion website at www.ataglanceseries.com/TandO to test yourself on these topics.

35 General principles 1

Figure 35.1 Fracture mechanisms
The type and direction of the force determines fracture pattern. High-energy mechanisms result in comminution

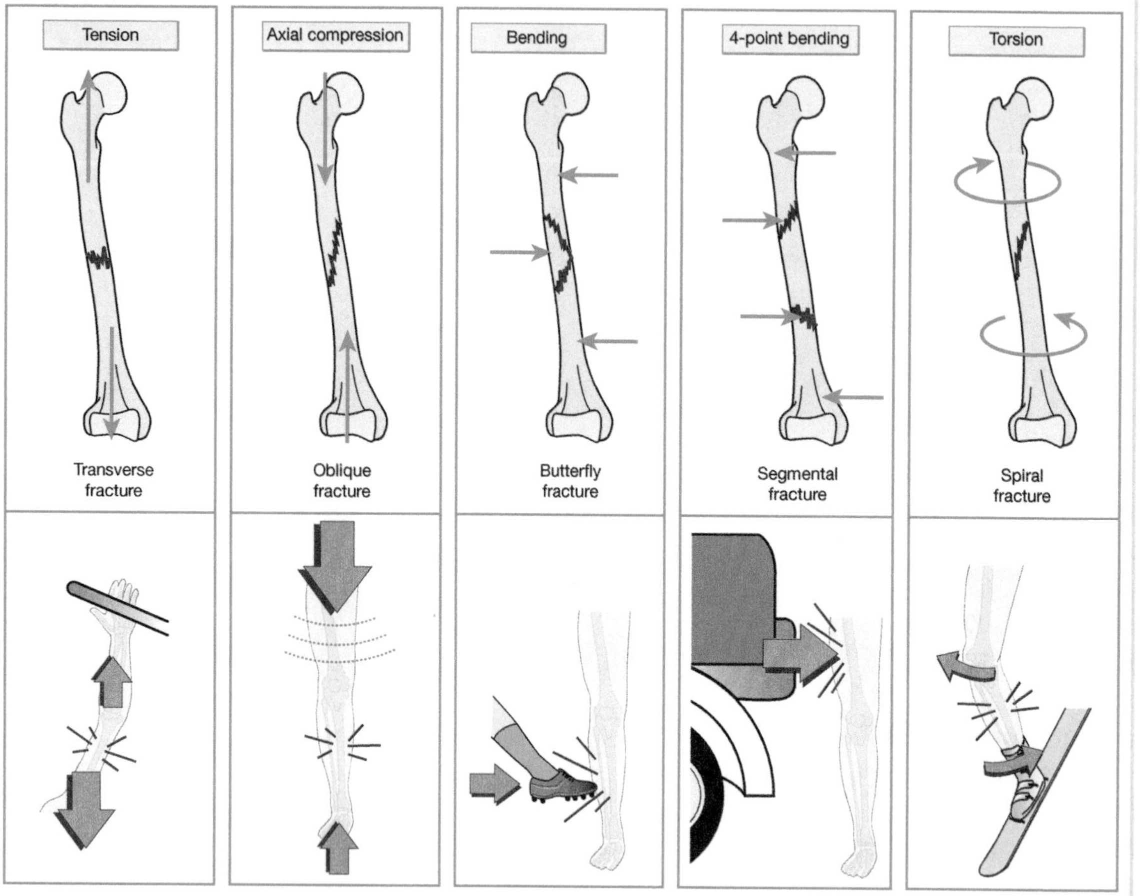

Tension	Axial compression	Bending	4-point bending	Torsion

Transverse fracture	Oblique fracture	Butterfly fracture	Segmental fracture	Spiral fracture

Figure 35.2 Gustilo and Anderson classification of open fractures

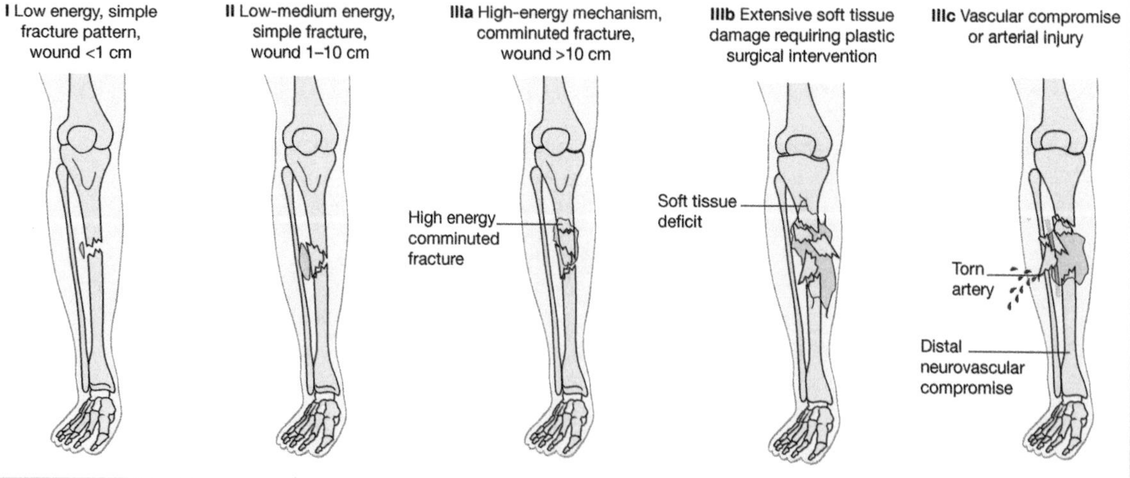

I Low energy, simple fracture pattern, wound <1 cm

II Low-medium energy, simple fracture, wound 1–10 cm

IIIa High-energy mechanism, comminuted fracture, wound >10 cm

High energy comminuted fracture

IIIb Extensive soft tissue damage requiring plastic surgical intervention

Soft tissue deficit

IIIc Vascular compromise or arterial injury

Torn artery

Distal neurovascular compromise

Fracture patterns

A fracture is a breech in the cortex of a bone. It is caused by the application of energy to the skeleton. There are two things that determine the type of fracture that results: the amount of energy and the way in which it is applied.

Mode of energy application

- Tension results in a transverse fracture.
- Axial compression results in an oblique fracture.
- Bending is a combination of tension and compression: as the bone is bent, the concave side is compressed whereas the convex side is put under tension. The result is an oblique fracture. Often there are two oblique fractures, which combine to make a triangular butterfly fragment.

Trauma and Orthopaedics at a Glance, First Edition. Henry Willmott.
© 2016 John Wiley & Sons, Ltd. Published 2016 by John Wiley & Sons, Ltd. Companion website: www.ataglanceseries.com/TandO

- If a bone is struck by a large rigid object, such as a car bumper, four-point bending forces may be generated. This results in a segmental fracture.
- Twisting or 'torsion' results in a spiral fracture, which may extend the full length of the bone.

There are a few other important fracture types:
- Avulsion fractures occur when a strong ligament or tendon is pulled off the bone with a fragment of bone.
- Greenstick and buckle fractures are incomplete fractures occurring in children; they are discussed in Chapter 48.
- Pathological fractures occur after a level of trauma that would not normally be expected to result in fracture, such as a fall from standing height. They may be due to osteoporosis or tumour.
- Stress fractures occur after repeated minor trauma and are a result of damage accumulation within the bone. They are often seen in individuals undergoing military or athletic training. Tiny hairline fractures occur in the metatarsals of the foot, for example, but the patient does not rest to allow healing to occur. Repeated loading of the bone results in an ongoing attempted healing response.

Amount of energy

In order to generate a fracture, energy must be applied to the bone in the form of kinetic energy generated either by an object colliding with the body, or the body colliding with a stationary object, most commonly the ground!

Kinetic energy is defined as $E = \frac{1}{2}mv^2$. Faster-moving or heavier objects colliding with the body, or a fall from a greater height in a heavier patient, results in larger amounts of energy imparted to the skeleton.

Greater energy results in more complicated fracture patterns, greater injury to the surrounding soft tissues, involvement of multiple bones and sometimes injury to other organs or systems. The complexity of the fracture pattern, and the degree of fragmentation is referred to as **comminution**.

If a patient has a highly comminuted fracture, there has been a large amount of energy involved. This is of paramount clinical importance. Comminuted fractures are at high risk for:
- associated visceral injuries;
- soft-tissue injury and subsequent compartment syndrome or neurovascular deficit;
- stripping of periosteum, which compromises the blood supply to fracture fragments and increases the risk of non-union.

Description

When describing a fracture, use the acronym **PARTS**:
- **Pattern**: transverse, spiral, oblique, butterfly, comminuted.

Next, describe the **displacement** of a fracture. Displacement is described with reference to the movement of the distal part relative to the proximal part. There are four ways a fracture can be displaced:
- **Angulation**: varus or valgus, anterior or posterior.
- **Rotation**: only properly appreciated on an X-ray showing the joint above and the joint below the fracture.
- **Translation**: movement of distal fracture fragment anteriorly or posteriorly, laterally or medially.
- **Shortening**: due to pull of muscles (it is rare for a fracture to be lengthened).

Open fractures
Definition

When a fracture occurs, a haematoma forms around the broken bone ends. If the fracture haematoma communicates with an epithelialised surface, it is an open fracture. An open fracture does not always communicate with the skin. Pelvic fractures may communicate with the rectum or vagina; maxillofacial fractures may communicate with the buccal cavity. In addition, the bone ends themselves do not have to protrude through the epithelialised surface – a laceration that is continuous with the haematoma constitutes an open fracture.

Sometimes it is difficult to decide if a small puncture wound communicates with fracture haematoma. One sign that is often helpful is the presence of continuous slow venous bleeding. In any event, it is important to have a high index of suspicion. If you think that it might be an open fracture, it probably is and should be treated as such.

Classification

Open fractures are described by the **Gustilo and Anderson classification**. It is based on the amount of energy of the injury, the degree of soft-tissue damage and the presence of vascular compromise. See figure 35.2.

Problems associated with open fractures
Early problems

The large amount of energy required to produce an open fracture, especially type III fractures, puts the patient at risk of:
- multi-system injury;
- compartment syndrome;
- nerve or vessel injury.

Later problems
- Infection – exposure of the fracture to the outside environment. The presence of crushed or devitalised tissue further increases this risk. Early administration of antibiotics and thorough debridement is key.
- Periosteal stripping and non-union – the bone relies on the periosteum to provide a blood supply for healing. It this is stripped, risk of non-union is high.

Treatment and the BOA guidelines

The British Orthopaedic Association (BOA) has published guidelines for the management of open tibial fractures. They are available at http://www.boa.ac.uk/Publications/Pages/BOASTs.aspx.

The principles are relevant to the management of all open fractures:

1 Initial assessment in accordance with advanced trauma life support (ATLS) principles and simultaneous management of associated injuries.

2 Careful assessment of the limb neurovascular status with clear documentation before and after manipulation. If vascular injury is suspected seek vascular opinion.

3 Remove gross contamination from the wound, photograph, and cover with a saline-soaked gauze and an impermeable membrane such as clingfilm. Avoid repeated exposure of the wound. Avoid provisional cleaning in A&E.

4 If the fracture is grossly displaced, restore alignment and then splint using a backslab.

5 Antibiotics and tetanus – Co-amoxiclav or cefuroxime and gentamicin are recommended.

6 Obtain X-rays: two views of the bone, including the joints above and below.

7 Assess for presence of compartment syndrome.

8 Wound debridement should be performed in theatre by a senior surgeon on a scheduled operating list in daylight hours within 24 hours of injury. Indications for immediate surgery are gross contamination, compartment syndrome or vascular compromise.

9 Primary amputation may be considered if the limb has been avascular for more than 6 hours, there is segmental muscle or bone loss.

10 Make an early referral to a specialist centre if the appropriate expertise is not available locally.

36 **General principles 2**

Figure 36.1 Fracture healing

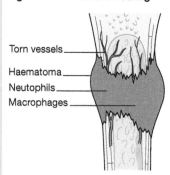
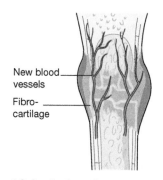
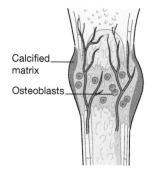
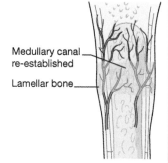

Torn vessels

Haematoma

Neutophils

Macrophages

New blood vessels

Fibro-cartilage

Calcified matrix

Osteoblasts

Medullary canal re-established

Lamellar bone

1 Haematoma formation:
Damage blood vessels bleed and result in a haematoma. Neutrophils secrete signalling molecules which recruit macrophages

2 Soft callus formation:
Collagen and fibrocartilage bridge the fracture site and new blood vessels form

3 Hard callus formation:
Osteoblasts, brought in by the new blood vessels, mineralise the fibrocartilage to produce woven bone

4 Remodelling:
Over months to years, osteoclasts remove woven bone and osteoblasts lay down ordered lamellar bone

Figure 36.2 Primary bone healing
If fracture is held with absolute stability and direct apposition of bone ends without a gap, primary bone healing may occur. Cutting cones are comprised of osteoclasts, which burrow a tunnel across the fracture site, followed by osteoblasts which lay down lamellar bone in the wake of the cutting cone. No callus is produced

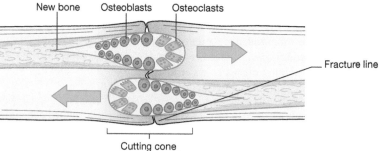

New bone   Osteoblasts   Osteoclasts

Fracture line

Cutting cone

Figure 36.3 Fracture treatment options

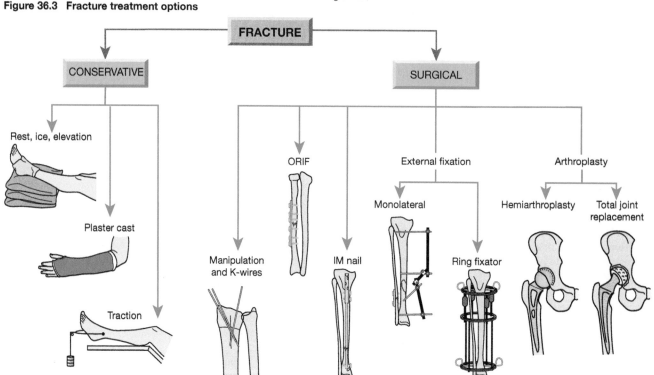

FRACTURE

CONSERVATIVE

SURGICAL

Rest, ice, elevation

Plaster cast

Traction

ORIF

Manipulation and K-wires

IM nail

External fixation

Monolateral

Ring fixator

Arthroplasty

Hemiarthroplasty

Total joint replacement

Trauma and Orthopaedics at a Glance, First Edition. Henry Willmott.
© 2016 John Wiley & Sons, Ltd. Published 2016 by John Wiley & Sons, Ltd. Companion website: www.ataglanceseries.com/TandO

Fracture healing

Fractures heal in four stages. Although each is considered as a separate stage, in reality they are a continuum:

- **Haematoma and inflammation** – bleeding from the broken edges of the bone results in a haematoma. Neutrophils secrete cytokines. Macrophages are recruited to remove dead tissue. Fibroblasts then lay down granulation tissue.
- **Soft callus** – within 2 weeks, collagen bridges the fracture site. The collagen is unmineralised and soft, and provides little structural support.
- **Hard callus** – after around 6 weeks, the soft callus becomes mineralised. Osteoblasts lay down hydroxyapatite and the callus becomes stiffer and stronger. It is poorly organised and bulky and can be seen on X-ray as fluffy calcification.
- **Remodelling** – over months and years, the poorly organised hard callus is resorbed and in its place strong lamellar bone is laid down.

This process is known as **secondary bone healing**, and it occurs in the presence of *micromovement* between fracture fragments. Tiny amounts of movement, in the order of micrometres, stimulate the various cells to become active and produce callus. This is known as **relative stability**.

Excessive movement results in disruption of the soft callus, and the result is non-union.

Primary bone healing

Bone may heal in another way, known as **primary bone healing**. In order for it to occur, there are two prerequisites:

- The bone ends must be absolutely stable, with no micromovement.
- The bone ends must be in direct apposition with no gap.

These conditions are known as **absolute stability** and it is achieved if a fracture is plated and compressed (see below).

Primary fracture healing occurs without the formation of callus. Osteoclasts drill tunnels directly across the fracture site. In their wake osteoblasts follow, laying down layers of strong, organised lamellar bone.

Fracture treatment options

In general, the treatment of all fractures can be summarised by the mantra **reduce, hold, rehabilitate**.

What constitutes an acceptable reduction depends on:

- **The site of the fracture** – if a joint surface is involved, anatomical reduction must be achieved to prevent arthritis.
- **The age of the patient** – children have huge potential to remodel.
- **Functional demands of the patient** – the required level of function and specific hobbies or sports may dictate what is acceptable to the patient.

There are many ways of holding the fracture in position whilst it heals:

- *Rest* – many fractures may be successfully treated with nothing more than a few weeks of rest. Examples include small avulsion fractures or stress fractures. The patient may be provided with crutches or a splint.
- *Traction* – application of traction to a limb uses gravity to keep the limb in alignment. This method has largely fallen out of favour because it involves a prolonged hospital stay, but traction still has a role in the temporary stabilisation of fractures awaiting surgical intervention and in the management of fractures in very young children who produce large amounts of callus within a couple of weeks.
- *Plaster cast* – a plaster cast provides relative stability allowing secondary fracture healing. Application of plaster is a skill that requires practice. Too little padding results in pressure sores, too much padding allows excessive fracture movement. A plaster that is too tight can cause compartment syndrome. For the first week after injury a backslab (half plaster, half bandage) allows swelling of an acutely injured limb.
- *K-wires* – simple fractures that remain unstable despite closed reduction may be held with percutaneous Kirschner wires. These sharp-tipped wires are passed through small stab incisions. The wires are left protruding through the skin to be removed after 4 weeks.
- *ORIF* – open reduction and internal fixation. Fractures that cannot be adequately reduced by manipulation need to be reduced by direct manipulation of the fracture fragments. Stability is then maintained by application of a plate and screws. If the fracture is reduced anatomically and compression applied between fracture fragments, absolute stability is provided, resulting in primary fracture healing. This method is therefore suitable for fractures extending into a joint.
- *IM nail* – long-bone fractures can be stabilised by passing a metal rod into the medullary canal. This is known as intramedullary nailing. It provides relative stability.
- *External fixator* – if a fracture is highly comminuted such that anatomical reduction cannot be achieved, if an open fracture is heavily contaminated or the soft tissues are grossly swollen such that wound healing may be compromised, an external fixator can be applied. The fixator is akin to scaffolding on a building. The fixation is outside the body, and the bone is held in place with pins passing through small stab incisions. A circular frame is a highly stable type of external fixator and instead of pins, tiny wires hold the bone fragments in place.
- *Arthroplasty* – if the blood supply to the fracture has been compromised, or the fracture is highly comminuted and extends into a joint, joint replacement may be considered. Examples include intracapsular hip fractures and comminuted proximal humerus fractures.

Choice of treatment option

There are many fixation options available and it may seem difficult at first to choose the correct one. Each patient is different, and each fracture is different. There is often more than one option – which is why trauma meetings may sometimes become animated!

In principle, though, for every fracture consider:

- **The personality of the patient** – what is their functional level, what are their demands, do medical comorbidities preclude surgery, will they cooperate with postoperative instructions, will they tolerate non-weightbearing on crutches?
- **The personality of the fracture** – what is the bone quality like, does the fracture involve a joint surface, how stable is the fracture, is it likely to displace?

37 Advanced trauma life support (ATLS)

Figure 37.1 ATLS primary survey

		Assess	Diagnosis	Intervention
A	Airway and cervical spine control	In-line immobilisation Talking? Look, listen, feel	Apnoea Airway obstruction	Collar Airway manoeuvres Air adjuncts Intubation
B	Breathing	Breathing pattern Oxygen saturation ABG	Apnoea Haemothorax Tension pneumothorax Open pneumothorax Flail chest	O_2 Needle thoracocentesis Chest drain Mechanical ventilation
C	Circulation and haemorrage control	BP HR Capillary refill Skin colour	Bleeding into thorax, abdomen, pelvis, thighs, external	IV cannulae Fluid bolus FAST scan Surgical assessment CT if stable
D	Disability and neurological function	GCS Pupillary reaction Limb movement	Intracerebral bleed Spinal injury	CT head Neurological assessment
E	Exposure and environmental control	Log roll Spinal tenderness or step PR examination Core temperature	Spinal injury Hypothermia	X-ray, CT Warming blanket

Assess systematically, identify and treat pathology as it is found.
If the situation changes, go back to A and reassess

Advanced trauma life support (ATLS)

A framework for the management of acute trauma, ATLS was developed in 1976 by an American orthopaedic surgeon, James Styner, who crashed his light aircraft in a remote part of Nebraska. His wife was killed instantly and his four children sustained major injuries. The treatment they received at the local hospital was so poor that he felt medical training needed to change. The ATLS system was adopted by the American College of Surgeons in 1980 and is now widely used around the world.

The core principles of ATLS are:
• Rapid evaluation of the trauma patient in a systematic method.
• Establishing management priorities – things that will kill the patient first are detected and treated first.
• Instigating treatment as injuries are found.

The 'golden hour'

The first hour after a major injury is a crucial time for the patient. Deaths after trauma occur in three peaks:
• Seconds to minutes after the injury – some injuries are unsurvivable. Massive head trauma, avulsion of the aorta due to rapid deceleration, or catastrophic external haemorrhage kill patients immediately or within a few minutes.
• Within an hour of the injury – known as the 'golden hour'. Injuries such as tension pneumothorax, haemorrhage due to unstable pelvic fractures and brain injury due to expanding intracranial haematoma kill patients within an hour. Recognition and treatment of these injuries will save lives. This is the *raison d'être* of ATLS.

• Days or weeks after injury – often due to infection or organ dysfunction, many of these late deaths can be avoided by good orthopaedic and surgical care in hospital.

Primary survey

On arrival, the trauma patient should be evaluated using ABDCE:

Airway and cervical spine protection

Talk to the patient – do they respond? If so, they probably have a patent airway and are oxygenating their brain. Noisy breathing or apnoea may indicate airway obstruction. Vigorous manoeuvres such as a head tilt may damage the spinal cord if there is a spine fracture and should be avoided. Protect the cervical spine with a collar, sand bags and tape to hold the head still. Open the airway with a jaw thrust or chin lift. If the airway is still compromised, adjuncts such as a Guedel airway or nasopharyngeal tube may help. If the patient has a decreased level of consciousness, they must be intubated using a cuffed endotracheal tube.

Breathing and oxygenation

Once the airway is secure, assess the breathing. Breathing is a combination of ventilation and oxygenation.

Administer oxygen at 15 L/min.

Assess the adequacy of ventilation by watching the breathing pattern, auscultating the chest, percussing the thorax and examining the position of the trachea. A pulse oximeter measures oxygen saturation although this may be misleading in the presence of carbon monoxide poisoning after a house fire, for example.

Trauma and Orthopaedics at a Glance, First Edition. Henry Willmott.
© 2016 John Wiley & Sons, Ltd. Published 2016 by John Wiley & Sons, Ltd. Companion website: www.ataglanceseries.com/TandO

- **Apnoea** requires mechanical ventilation.
- Unilateral absent breath sounds and a dull percussion note indicate a **haemothorax**, which must be drained with a chest drain.
- Unilateral absent breath sounds and a hyperresonant percussion note indicate a **pneumothorax**, which must be drained with a chest drain.
- A pneumothorax with tracheal deviation indicates a **tension pneumothorax** whereby a one-way valve effect results in a build-up of air under pressure between the chest wall and the lung. This reduces venous return as well as oxygenation and can kill a patient very rapidly. Treat by relieving the pressure with a grey cannula placed in the second intercostal space, followed by a chest drain.
- A wound to the chest may result in an **open pneumothorax** whereby air is entrained preferentially through a large chest wall defect rather than into the lungs. Cover the wound with an occlusive dressing, taping down three sides only so that it acts like a valve, allowing air out but not in. Then place a chest drain.
- A **flail chest** is multiple rib fractures resulting in a segment of chest wall that moves independently of the rest of the thorax. As the patient inspires, the flail segment does not move with the rest of the ribs, resulting in hypoventilation. The result is hypoxia and the patient rapidly fatigues. The treatment is mechanical ventilation to support the patient's respiratory efforts.

Circulation and haemorrhage control

Only after A and B have been addressed do you move on to C. All patients require two large-bore cannulae. At the same time, take blood including a specimen for cross-match. Two litres of warmed Hartmann's solution should be administered.

Adequacy of circulation is assessed by blood pressure, pulse rate and volume. Central capillary refill, measured by pressing on the sternum, and skin temperature are also useful.

Haemorrhage can occur in five places:
- **The thorax** – haemothorax may result in hypovolaemia. Penetrating injuries to the heart may result in cardiac tamponade whereby blood accumulates between the pericardium and the myocardium, restricting cardiac output. Treatment of both these conditions requires the input of cardiothoracic surgeons.
- **The abdomen** – visceral injuries such as liver lacerations, spleen fracture or avulsion of bowel from its mesentery result in intra-abdominal bleeding and peritonism. Treatment is by laparotomy.
- **The pelvis** – when the pelvis is fractured, multiple vascular structures may be torn resulting in large amounts of bleeding. If the pelvis fracture is displaced, the volume of the pelvic cavity may be enlarged, leading to unabated continued haemorrhage. Assess the pelvis by looking for asymmetry, leg length discrepancy, perineal bruising or bleeding from the urethral meatus or vagina. Pelvic X-ray confirms the diagnosis. The treatment is to apply a tight strap around the hips to pull the two halves of the pelvis back together. This can be done with a bed sheet or a pelvic binder. Although application of a binder may result in tamponade, surgery is normally required to fix the pelvis and repair or tie-off bleeding vessels.
- **The thighs** – fractured femurs can bleed heavily. Evaluate the femurs by looking for deformity and feeling for swelling and crepitus. Treatment is initially traction to align the bone, restrict movement and reduce pain. Surgical fixation is usually required.
- **The floor** – always check the floor for a puddle of blood – wounds bleed! If left unchecked, hypovolaemia will result. Treat with direct pressure initially, followed by formal exploration and closure.

Assess response to the fluid bolus frequently. If shock is on-going, re-evaluate for potential sources of haemorrhage.

Disability

Assessment of cerebral function is next. Measure the Glasgow Coma Score (GCS) and pupillary response.

EYE OPENING	VERBAL	MOTOR
4 – spontaneous	5 – normal	6 – normal
3 – to voice	4 – disorientated	5 – localises pain
2 – to pain	3 – incoherent words	4 – withdraws from pain
1 – none	2 – incomprehensible sounds	3 – abnormal flexion
		2 – abnormal extension
	1 – none	1 – none

Although the patient may be drunk or under the influence of drugs, could the reduced GCS be a result of intracranial haemorrhage due to a head injury? A CT scan of the head should be performed if in doubt. Reduced GCS may result in airway compromise. If GCS is less than 8, the patient should be intubated.

Exposure and environmental control

Expose the patient fully, removing all clothing to assess for occult injuries. Then examine the patient's back. In order to protect the spine, the patient should be carefully rolled to the side, maintaining alignment of the spinal column by means of a **log roll**. This needs three people to roll, one to support the head and neck, and one to examine the spine and back. Palpate the whole spine, feeling for crepitus, deformity or a step and assessing for pain. Finally, perform a rectal examination, checking sensation, tone and the presence of blood.

Once the log roll is complete, warm the patient using a warmer and blankets. Hypothermia is common in trauma patients.

Secondary survey

Once the primary survey has been completed and immediate life-threatening injuries treated or excluded, any other injuries should be identified. Examine the patient from top-to-toe, assessing for pain, deformity or loss of function. Although minor orthopaedic injuries will not kill the patient, functional outcome will suffer if they are not detected and treated appropriately.

This chapter is not a substitute for attending an ATLS course. The course is over 3 days and involves theory and practical teaching, culminating in a very realistic simulated-trauma practical exam. Most attendees agree it is a useful and enjoyable course.

38 Upper limb trauma 1

Figure 38.1 Clavicle fractures

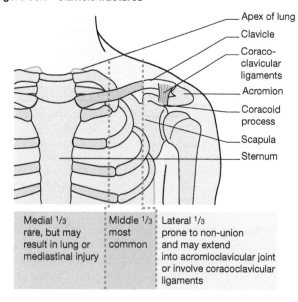

- Apex of lung
- Clavicle
- Coraco-clavicular ligaments
- Acromion
- Coracoid process
- Scapula
- Sternum

Medial ⅓ rare, but may result in lung or mediastinal injury	Middle ⅓ most common	Lateral ⅓ prone to non-union and may extend into acromioclavicular joint or involve coracoclavicular ligaments

Figure 38.2 AP X-ray of middle-third clavicle fracture showing a butterfly fragment, angulation and displacement of the fragments, but no significant shortening. This was managed conservatively

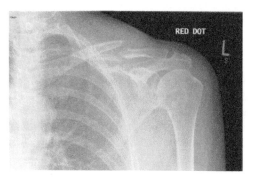

Figure 38.3 X-rays of normal shoulder
(a) AP view (b) Axillary view-note that the humeral head is seen sitting concentrically in the glenoid

(a)   (a)

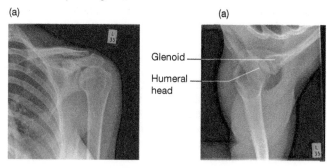

- Glenoid
- Humeral head

Figure 38.4 Anterior dislocation of the shoulder

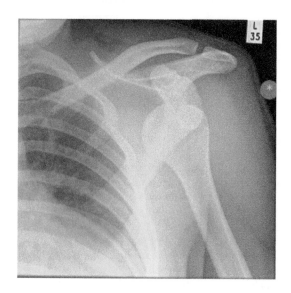

Figure 38.5 Proximal humerus fractures
Increasing force results in increased comminution of the proximal humerus. Surgical neck fractures may be treated conservatively in a collar and cuff; greater tuberosity fractures may need ORIF if they are displaced; 3-part fractures commonly need ORIF with a plate and screws; 4-part fractures may be fixed with ORIF, but if highly comminuted or displaced, hemiarthroplasty may be required

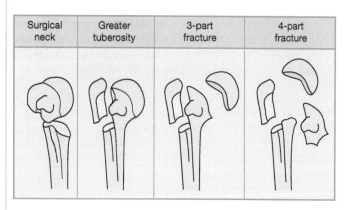

Surgical neck	Greater tuberosity	3-part fracture	4-part fracture

Figure 38.6 Undisplaced humerus surgical neck fracture

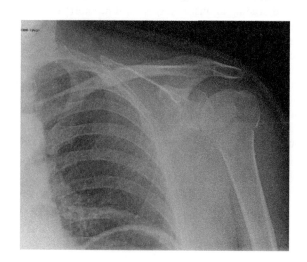

Trauma and Orthopaedics at a Glance, First Edition. Henry Willmott.
© 2016 John Wiley & Sons, Ltd. Published 2016 by John Wiley & Sons, Ltd. Companion website: www.ataglanceseries.com/TandO

Clavicle fractures

Clavicle fractures are common after a fall onto the shoulder. The clavicle lies directly over the brachial plexus, the subclavian artery and vein, and the apex of the lung. Any of these structures may be injured, and careful neurovascular examination and chest auscultation is important.

Fractures of the middle third are the most common, accounting for over 80% of cases. Lateral third fractures account for 15%, with medial third fractures around 5%. However, lateral third fractures have a higher risk of non-union, and medial third a higher risk of brachial plexus or lung injury.

X-rays should include an AP view and a 30° cephalad (tilted towards the head) view. The latter view prevents the ribs overlapping the clavicle.

Most cases can be managed conservatively with a collar and cuff for 4–6 weeks and mobilisation as tolerated. Absolute indications for surgery include open fractures, tenting or compromise of the skin or neurovascular injury. In addition, lateral third fractures may be managed surgically due to the high risk of non-union, especially if they extend into the acromioclavicular joint.

Fractures that are highly comminuted or have occurred as a result of a very high-energy mechanism have an increased risk of non-union and many surgeons opt to treat these surgically. If the fracture fragments have more than 2 cm overlap, the resultant shortening of the clavicle may reduce function of the shoulder and this is therefore a relative indication for surgery, although this point is controversial.

Shoulder dislocation

The shoulder joint is very shallow and relies heavily on the rotator cuff muscles and the cartilage lip around the glenoid for its stability. It is therefore relatively easy to dislocate. There are three types of dislocation, described by the direction the humeral head has moved:

- anterior – by far the commonest type (90%);
- posterior – associated with epileptic seizures and electric shocks;
- inferior – very rare, but easily recognised as the patient presents with the arm abducted above the head.

The patient presents with pain, restricted movement and loss of the normal shoulder contour. Clinical assessment should include examination of pulses and the brachial plexus, especially the integrity of the axillary nerve, which may be damaged as it runs around the neck of the humerus. The best way to test the axillary nerve is to assess sensation over the deltoid 'regimental badge' area.

X-ray evaluation is essential prior to any attempt at manipulation as fractures may be present – either of the humeral neck, the glenoid or avulsion of the greater tuberosity. At least two views are required – an AP and either an axillary or a scapular-Y (see Figure 38.2).

There are numerous techniques to reduce a dislocation. Vigorous manipulation or twisting may cause a humeral fracture and must be avoided. The first step is to ensure the patient is adequately relaxed. This can be achieved with Entonox® or small doses of opiates and benzodiazepines. **Extreme** caution must be exercised when administering these drugs, especially in the elderly. The patient must be monitored and given oxygen. Always seek senior support or ask an anaesthetist to help. The Hippocratic method is the safest manoeuvre: apply counter-traction in the axilla, traditionally applied with your foot; it is better to use a rolled sheet and the assistance of a nurse. Gentle in-line traction is applied to the arm. Gentle internal and external rotation is sometimes needed to disimpact the humeral head. Reduction is achieved with a clunk. Apply a broad arm sling and obtain repeat X-rays. If this fails, manipulation under anaesthetic with fluoroscopy guidance is often needed. Chapter 55 has more details.

Shoulder dislocation may result in injury to the humeral head or glenoid. The glenoid can dig a divot out of the humeral head, known as a Hill–Sachs lesion. The glenoid rim may be chipped off, known as a Bankart lesion. These bony lesions are commoner in young patients and may result in recurrent dislocation.

The rotator cuff may be torn, resulting in weakness and pain. This is commoner in elderly patients.

Acute rotator cuff tear

The rotator cuff comprises four muscles: supraspinatus, infraspinatus, subscapularis and teres minor. Together they form a hood around the head of the humerus and act to abduct, internally rotate and externally rotate the shoulder. They also provide stability to the joint.

The tendons of the cuff muscles can be torn by forced movement of the arm or shoulder dislocation. An acute tear presents as new-onset weakness and pain. This in contrast to a chronic tear, which occurs in the elderly and is due to gradual degeneration of the tendons and may be associated with arthritis.

Examine all three movements of the cuff, looking for focal weakness, comparing with the opposite side. MRI or ultrasound scan confirms the diagnosis. Treatment is repair of the cuff tendons, which may be performed arthroscopically.

Proximal humerus fractures

Falling onto an outstretched hand may result in fracture to the proximal humerus, especially in the elderly in association with osteoporosis. Broadly speaking there are three types of fracture: an avulsion of the greater tuberosity caused by the pull of supraspinatus, fracture of the surgical neck of the humerus, and comminuted fractures in which the head and tuberosities are separated.

Isolated tuberosity fractures can be managed conservatively in a broad-arm sling if undisplaced. If they are displaced, they should be fixed and treated in the same way as a rotator cuff tear.

Minimally displaced surgical neck fractures may be treated conservatively in a collar and cuff. This type of sling is preferred because it allows the weight of the arm to maintain alignment. The patient should be warned not to lean on the affected arm as this will cause displacement. Significant displacement mandates surgical fixation with a plate and screws.

Comminuted fractures that involve the head of the humerus are more difficult to treat. If the head of the humerus is split, or the fragments are widely displaced, the fracture is at risk of non-union, avascular necrosis or late development of arthritis. In these cases, the fracture is either fixed with a plate and screws, or the whole head is replaced with a hemiarthroplasty. Stiffness is common after this injury.

39 Upper limb trauma 2

Figure 39.1 (a) Many fractures of the humerus are managed in a brace and collar and cuff. Gravity helps to reduce the fracture and maintain alignment, (b) The radial nerve runs in close proximity to the humerus and can become trapped in the fracture site or injured by a bone fragment. This results in wrist drop

(a)

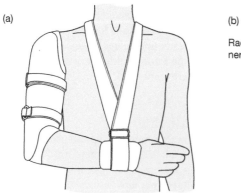

(b)

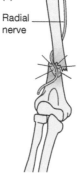

Radial nerve

Figure 39.2 (a) Olecranon fracture-there is a transverse fracture across the olecranon and the olecranon fragment has been pulled proximally by the triceps tendon. (b) Fixation of the olecranon fracture entailed open reduction and internal fixation using a technique known as 'tension band wiring'

(a)

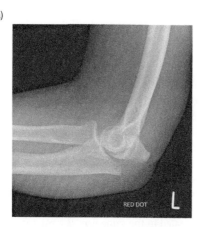

(b)

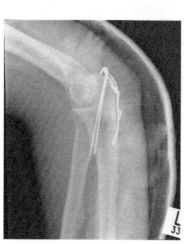

Figure 39.3 Galeazzi fracture
Fracture of the radius with dislocation of the distal radio-ulnar joint (a) The radial fracture is clearly demonstrated (b) The lateral shows dislocation of the DRUJ

(a)

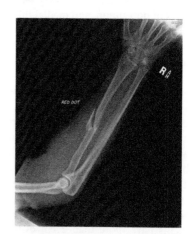

(b)

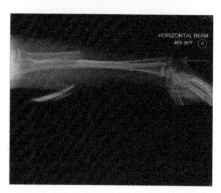

Figure 39.4 Monteggia fracture
Fracture of the proximal ulna with dislocation of the radiocapitellar joint. A line drawn along the length of the radius should normally intersect the middle third of the capitellum. Here, the radial head is dislocated posteriorly

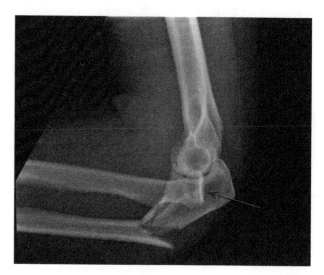

Trauma and Orthopaedics at a Glance, First Edition. Henry Willmott.
© 2016 John Wiley & Sons, Ltd. Published 2016 by John Wiley & Sons, Ltd. Companion website: www.ataglanceseries.com/TandO

Humeral shaft fractures

Fractures of the humerus are common, often caused by a direct blow to the arm resulting in a butterfly fragment, a twisting injury causing a spiral fracture, or a fall from standing in the elderly resulting in a transverse fracture.

Patients present with pain and deformity. Crepitus may be palpable.

Obtain AP and lateral X-rays and look carefully at the elbow and shoulder joints to ensure the fracture does not extend intra-articularly.

Radial nerve injury

Check carefully for radial nerve injury – the nerve runs closely apposed to the bone in the spiral groove and may be injured in up to 20% of cases. The radial nerve must be assessed on presentation and again after any splint or brace is applied. Test sensation in the anatomical snuff box and check power of wrist extension. Most radial nerve injuries are neuropraxia (bruising to the nerve), which resolves spontaneously and does not need surgery. If a nerve injury occurs after the fracture has been manipulated, there is a risk that the nerve might be trapped in the fracture site or lacerated by sharp bone fragments, and it should be explored surgically. Similarly, if a nerve fails to recover after 2–3 months, surgical exploration is indicated.

Treatment

Fracture treatment is most commonly non-surgical. A hanging cast or U-slab is applied for the first 2 weeks. A hanging cast adds weight to the distal arm to allow gravity to hold the fracture in alignment; a U-slab stabilises the fracture directly. Both are cumbersome and difficult to apply. Once swelling has subsided at around 2 weeks, the plaster can be removed and a functional brace applied. The brace is two rigid half-shells secured by Velcro straps. It must be applied tightly in order to squeeze the arm into alignment. Union can be expected in around 8 weeks.

Surgery is indicated in open fractures, vascular injury, new radial nerve injury after manipulation, in the context of multiple injuries, segmental fractures and pathological fractures. Surgical options include open reduction and internal fixation with a plate and screws, or intramedullary nailing.

Fractures around the elbow

The elbow is a modified hinge joint allowing flexion-extension and pronation-supination. The three bones involved are the humerus, the ulna and the radius.

Distal humerus

The distal humerus is composed of medial and lateral condyles. Fractures of the condyles may occur after a fall onto the arm. As with all joints, perfect anatomical alignment is essential for the elbow to remain functional. Condylar fractures are therefore normally treated with open reduction and internal fixation, usually using specially designed plates.

Proximal ulna (olecranon and coranoid)

The ulnar articulation of the elbow has a deep 'C' shape.

Posteriorly the olecranon provides insertion for the triceps tendon. The olecranon can be fractured if the elbow is forcibly flexed in a fall. A direct blow to the olecranon can also cause a fracture. It must be fixed to allow the triceps to function. The usual method is either wire fixation ('tension-band wiring') or plate fixation if the fracture is comminuted.

Anteriorly, the coronoid is a spike of bone that is an important stabiliser of the elbow, providing attachment for the capsular-ligamentous structures that prevent dislocation. The coronoid may be fractured if the elbow is dislocated. Fixation may be required to stabilise the joint.

Proximal radius

The radius articulates with the elbow at the radial head. This mushroom-shaped piece of bone rotates as the forearm is pronated and supinated. It abuts the capitellum of the humerus and provides stability to valgus stress. It may be fractured in a fall onto an outstretched hand or in an elbow dislocation. Generally speaking, if the fracture fragments are displaced less than 2 mm, no specific treatment is required other than analgesia and a sling for a couple of weeks. Significant displacement, comminution or instability of the elbow may require fixation or replacement with an artificial radial head.

Forearm fractures

The forearm is commonly fractured after a fall or a direct blow. The limb is composed of the radius and ulna. In order to pronate and supinate, the two bones must twist around one another. In order to maintain this action, length and alignment must be restored after a fracture.

Careful examination of neurovascular status is essential. The median, radial and ulnar nerves can all be damaged. Check radial and ulnar pulses and perform Allen's test. Swelling can sometimes be considerable and compartment syndrome may result. The ulna is subcutaneous and open fractures are therefore relatively common.

Both bone fractures

If both radius and ulna are fractured, alignment must be restored and maintained. Undisplaced fractures may be managed conservatively in an above-elbow cast. Displacement is usually an indication for surgery. In adults, open reduction and internal fixation with plates and screws is preferred.

Nightstick fracture

Isolated ulnar fractures may occur after a direct blow to the ulna border of the forearm. This is a common defensive injury if an assailant wields a heavy weapon at an individual. They are known as nightstick fractures, following notorious American police brutality in the Prohibition era. Although alignment may be maintained, non-union risk is high, and these fractures are normally treated by ORIF with plate and screws.

Galeazzi fracture

Isolated fracture of the distal radius shaft with disruption of the distal-radio-ulnar joint (DRUJ) is known as a Galeazzi fracture. The DRUJ is assessed on a true lateral X-ray. Dorsal displacement and tenderness suggest that it is injured. The radius must be fixed with ORIF and plate, and the DRUJ stability assessed intraoperatively. Persistent instability mandates temporary K-wire fixation to hold it reduced.

Monteggia fracture

An isolated proximal third ulnar fracture with dislocation of the radial head is called a Monteggia fracture. The radial head should be aligned with the capitellum, and on an elbow X-ray (AP or lateral) a line drawn up the shaft of the radius should transect the middle of the capitellum (known as the radiocapitellar line). Reduction and fixation of the ulnar fracture usually restores alignment of the radiocapitellar joint.

40 Upper limb trauma 3

Figure 40.1 Normal angulation of the distal radius

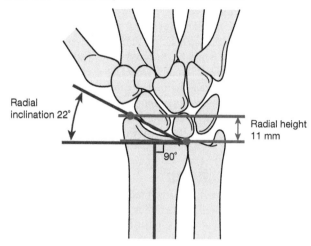

Radial inclination 22°

Radial height 11 mm

90°

Volar tilt 11°

90°

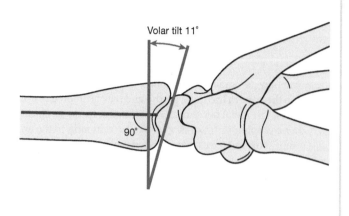

Figure 40.2 X-ray of distal radius fracture
(a) AP (b) lateral

(a)

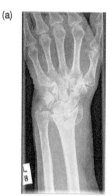

(b)

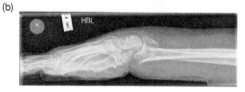

HBL

Figure 40.3 Fixation of intra-articular distal radius fracture
The plate has been used to reconstruct the articular surface and restore alignment. (a) AP (b) lateral

(a)   (b)

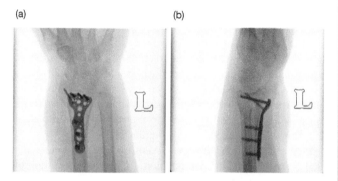

Figure 40.5 Mallet finger
The extensor tendon has been avulsed from the distal phalynx. A fragment of bone is sometimes pulled off

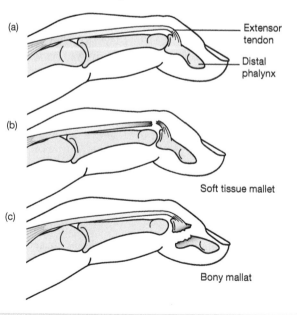

(a) Extensor tendon / Distal phalynx

(b) Soft tissue mallet

(c) Bony mallat

Figure 40.4 Perilunate dislocation
This injury is sometimes missed because it is not immediately obvious on the (a) AP view. The (b) lateral view shows the capitate has dislocated dorsally, although the lunate remains congruent with the distal radius

(a)   (b)

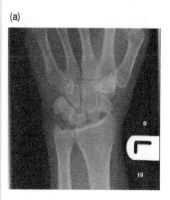

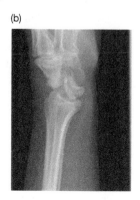

Trauma and Orthopaedics at a Glance, First Edition. Henry Willmott.
© 2016 John Wiley & Sons, Ltd. Published 2016 by John Wiley & Sons, Ltd. Companion website: www.ataglanceseries.com/TandO

Distal radius fractures

These are extremely common, affecting both young and elderly patients. The usual mechanism is a fall onto an outstretched hand.

Anatomy

The end of the distal radius is concave and articulates with the scaphoid and lunate carpal bones, allowing extension and flexion of the wrist. The normal orientation of the joint surface is:
- 11° palmar tilt (also known as volar tilt; in sagittal plane);
- 22° radial inclination (in coronal plane);
- the radius is 11 mm longer than the ulna (radial length).

Patients present with pain and restricted movement at the wrist. There may be visible deformity. Check median and ulnar nerve function carefully as they run close to the bone here.

PA and lateral views should be obtained, assessing for displacement, angulation, comminution, shortening and extension into the joint.

The most common direction of displacement is dorsal after a fall onto the hand. Remember that the normal position of the joint surface is a 11° tilt towards the palm. Osteoporotic patients may have dorsal comminution, which makes the fracture unstable. High-energy mechanisms of injury increase the risk of intra-articular extension.

Eponymous names

Eponymous names have historically been used to describe specific fracture configurations. Often misused, their use is to be discouraged. They are listed here so that you can correct your colleagues when they get it wrong:
- Colles' – simple extra-articular transverse fracture of the distal radius one inch (2.5 cm) from the joint line with dorsal displacement and a 'dinner-fork deformity' (this was described before X-rays were discovered).
- Smith's – also known as a reverse Colles', an extra-articular fracture with palmar displacement.
- Barton's (volar or dorsal) – a partial intra-articular fracture in which either the dorsal or palmar rim of the radius is left intact.

Treatment

First, describe the fracture and assess displacement and intra-articular extension. Undisplaced extra-articular fractures may be managed conservatively in a below-elbow cast for a total of 6 weeks. The first week is in a backslab to allow for swelling.

Displaced fractures need reduction. If the fracture is extra-articular, closed reduction may be attempted. This may be performed under haematoma block (see Chapter 55). If reduction is satisfactory, a trial of conservative treatment in plaster is merited. It should be remembered that if a fracture requires manipulation, there is a risk of redisplacement. This risk is especially high if there is dorsal comminution. Close monitoring with weekly X-rays will detect displacement. If there is significant instability, K-wires may be used to hold the distal fragment in position.

Intra-articular fractures require anatomical reduction if arthritis is to be avoided. This may be achieved by ORIF using a plate and screws.

Carpal injury
Scaphoid fractures

There are eight carpal bones but the commonest one to be fractured is the scaphoid. The mechanism is usually a fall backwards onto the hand, forcing the wrist into extension. The patient complains of pain on the radial side of the wrist. Tenderness is maximal in the anatomical snuff box.

The scaphoid is difficult to visualise on X-ray because of overlap of the other carpal bones and the radial styloid. Request 'scaphoid views' – four views with the wrist in various positions. Fractures may be subtle. Trace the cortex looking for a breach. If the patient has a convincing clinical picture for scaphoid fracture but the X-rays look normal, it is quite reasonable to bring him or her back to fracture clinic in a week with a splint or plaster in the meantime. CT or MRI are much more sensitive.

The scaphoid has a retrograde blood supply. Displaced fractures may therefore disrupt the blood supply to the proximal pole of the scaphoid, resulting in non-union, avascular necrosis and eventually instability and arthritis. Displaced fractures are therefore treated with screw fixation.

Undisplaced fractures may be treated in plaster, but healing is slow, sometimes taking several months. Some surgeons therefore prefer to fix even undisplaced fractures. If plaster is to be used, a below-elbow cast is all that is required. The traditional 'scaphoid cast' incorporated the thumb, but studies have proven that a below-elbow plaster leaving the thumb free is just as good, and your patient will thank you for the extra function this allows!

Perilunate dislocation

This is a very rare injury, but one not to be missed. The carpal bones are in two rows. The distal row may become separated from the proximal row in a very high-energy injury such as a motorcycle crash. The lunate is sometimes extruded into the carpal tunnel, compressing the median nerve.

The hand is grossly swollen and there may be paraesthesia in the median nerve distribution. AP X-rays look unusual, but the injury cannot be clearly seen unless a true lateral is performed. If in doubt, obtain a lateral view, or a CT scan and reduce urgently.

Metacarpal fractures

Often caused by punching, look carefully for wounds over the knuckles, which may have been caused by the opponent's teeth. Risk of infection is high, and the wound should be washed out and antibiotics administered.

Rotation of the fracture causes 'scissoring' (crossing-over) of the finger and is poorly tolerated. Reduction and fixation with wires, screws or plate is indicated.

Mallet fractures

The dorsal rim of the distal phalanx is the insertion for the extensor tendon. Avulsion of the tendon results in a mallet finger. There is a characterisic droop.

Treatment is to splint the finger in extension. Repeat X-rays in the splint. Subluxation of the joint, or involvement of more than a third of the articular surface, is an indication for surgical fixation.

41 Lower limb trauma 1

Figure 41.1 Pelvic fractures

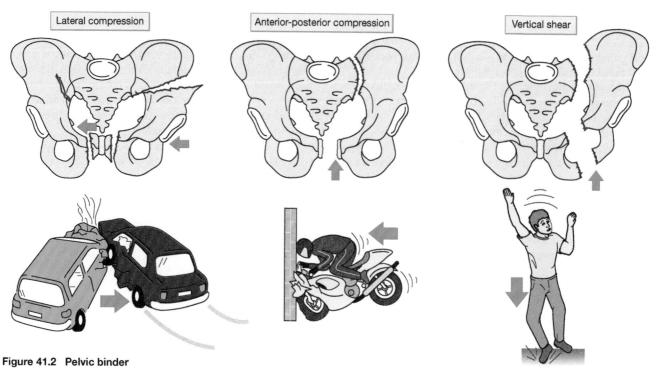

Lateral compression | Anterior-posterior compression | Vertical shear

Figure 41.2 Pelvic binder
The binder should be applied at the level of the greater trochanters in order to reduce pelvic volume and tamponade bleeding. A tightly applied sheet is an alternative if no binder is available.

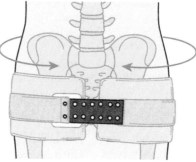

Figure 41.3 Acetabular fracture
Often associated with a hip dislocation, a posterior directed force may fracture the posterior wall of the acetabulum. The hip must be reduced urgently and the fracture fixed to restore the congruency of the joint

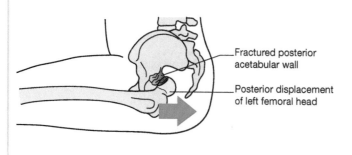

Fractured posterior acetabular wall

Posterior displacement of left femoral head

Figure 41.4 Femoral nail
The nail may be passed retrograde (from the knee), or antegrade from the greater trochanter

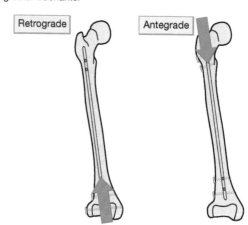

Retrograde | Antegrade

Trauma and Orthopaedics at a Glance, First Edition. Henry Willmott.
© 2016 John Wiley & Sons, Ltd. Published 2016 by John Wiley & Sons, Ltd. Companion website: www.ataglanceseries.com/TandO

Pelvic fractures

There are few fractures that can kill a patient within hours, but pelvic fractures fall into this category. The pelvis is surrounded by a rich plexus of blood vessels, which can be torn by fractured bone. Unlike the limbs, no tourniquet or direct pressure can be applied and the result may be fatal bleeding.

The pelvis is composed of two hemipelves or 'innominate bones' (made up of the fused pubis, ilium and ischium) and the sacrum. Posteriorly the sacrum connects to the innominate bones at the sacroiliac joints. Anteriorly the innominate bones are connected by the symphysis pubis.

Mechanism of injury

The pelvis is a stable construct and it takes a large amount of energy to fracture it. Therefore, the risk of associated visceral or musculoskeletal injuries is high. There are four types of pelvic fracture, described by the direction of causative force:

- **Lateral compression** – seen in side-swipe car accidents, one half of the pelvis is pushed inwards resulting in sacroiliac joint disruption or sacral fracture. Continued force pushes the contralateral side of the pelvis outwards.
- **Anterior-posterior compression** – seen in head-on collisions, particularly motorcyclists hitting the fuel tank of the bike; the pelvis springs open, hinging on the sacroiliac joints.
- **Vertical shear** – a fall from a height results in one hemipelvis being pushed upwards, shearing the sacrum posteriorly.
- **Combined** – combined force vectors cause a mixed picture.

Evaluation

Use the ATLS algorithm. Assess perineal bruising and leg length discrepancy. Palpate the iliac crests, feeling for asymmetry. Vigorous pushing on the iliac crests to assess stability is not recommended as it may worsen bleeding. An X-ray is essential. Special views can be obtained to visualise the anterior or posterior half of the pelvis, but in the context of acute trauma, a CT scan is quicker and gives more information.

Bone fragments may tear vagina, bladder, urethra or rectum. Perform a PR and PV examination. Look for blood at the urethral meatus. If urethral injury is suspected, a urethrogram should be performed.

Treatment

Stick to ATLS! Hypovolaemia is common. Obtain IV access, cross-match blood, resuscitate the patient. Application of a pelvic binder at the level of the greater trochanters may help to reduce the pelvic volume and tamponade bleeding. Haemodynamic instability mandates laparotomy or angiographic embolisation of bleeding vessels.

Definitive treatment is carried out in a specialist centre. The principle is to restore the integrity of the pelvic ring and alignment of the sacroiliac joints. Plates and screws are used. If a patient is too unstable for this invasive surgery, an external fixator may be applied.

Acetabular fractures

Forces applied through the leg may result in fracture of the acetabulum. A common mechanism is when the knee strikes the dashboard in a car accident. The hip is pushed backwards against the posterior wall of the acetabulum resulting in a fracture. The hip may also dislocate. If this is the case, the hip should be urgently reduced under anaesthetic to lessen the risk of avascular necrosis of the femoral head.

As with any fracture involving a joint, restoration of alignment is essential to avoid future arthritis. Open reduction and internal fixation may be achieved using a plate and screws. In older patients, a total hip replacement may be more suitable.

Fractures around the hip are discussed in Chapters 44 and 45.

Femoral shaft fractures

The femur is the largest bone in the body and it takes significant force to fracture it. There is therefore a high incidence of multiple injuries, and ATLS principles should be followed. Bleeding into the thigh may be significant. The elderly with osteoporosis or bone metastases can sustain femoral fractures with a low-energy mechanism. Such fractures are usually of spiral configuration.

Evaluation

Evaluation should include X-rays including images of the hip and knee. Look carefully to see if the fracture extends distally into the knee. Check distal pulses and neurological status. If surgery is likely, cross-match six units.

Treatment

Treatment is usually surgical, although definitive fixation may be delayed if the patient is unstable. An external fixator may be applied as an interim measure in this case.

Traction

Traction may be applied as a way of temporarily reducing pain and bleeding. The ambulance service use Thomas splints, devices that apply traction to the foot with counter-traction via a post in the groin. Although suitable for extraction and transportation, these devices should not be left in situ for more than a few hours due to the risk of perineal skin necrosis or pudendal nerve palsy. Instead, apply skin traction if the skin is otherwise healthy. Around 5 kg should be sufficient for most cases.

Intramedullary nailing

A nail stabilises the fracture without exposing the bone at the fracture site. This results in faster healing, less blood loss and smaller scars. The nail may be inserted from the proximal end of the bone (antegrade), or from the knee (retrograde). Antegrade nailing is most common. Retrograde nailing is indicated for very low femoral shaft fractures. It may also be used if a tibial fracture is being treated with a nail at the same time, so that both nails can be inserted through one incision.

Plate fixation

Open reduction and internal fixation with a plate is indicated for segmental fractures, in cases where the intramedullary canal is too narrow to pass a nail, in the presence of a hip replacement that is filling the canal, or if the fracture extends into the knee joint.

42 Lower limb trauma 2

Figure 42.1 Patella fracture

The patella may be fractured by a direct blow, resulting in a comminuted fracture, or by sudden contraction of the quadriceps against resistance, resulting in a transverse fracture

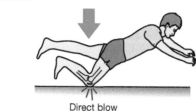

Direct blow

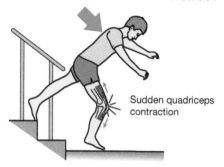

Sudden quadriceps contraction

Figure 42.3 Tibial plateau fractures: Schatzker classification

Lateral split	Lateral split and depression	Lateral depression
I	II	III
Medial	Both medial and lateral	Involvement of the metaphysis separating the joint surface from the shaft
IV	V	VI

Figure 42.2 Tension band wiring

Two parallel k-wires align the fracture fragments and compression is provided by a figure-of-eight wire under tension

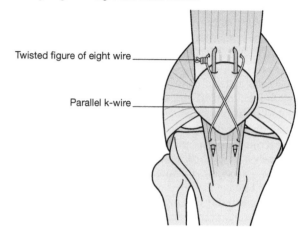

Twisted figure of eight wire

Parallel k-wire

Figure 42.4 (a) Tibial plateau fractures

AP and lateral x-rays of an oblique tibial fracture with a butterfly fragment. (a) The fracture is displace, shortened, in varus and recurvatum (apex posterior). There is an associated fibula fracture (b) The fracture was reduced and stabilised with a tibial nail

(a)

(b)

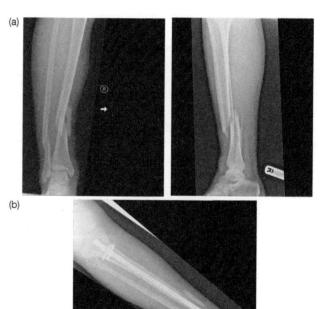

Trauma and Orthopaedics at a Glance, First Edition. Henry Willmott.
© 2016 John Wiley & Sons, Ltd. Published 2016 by John Wiley & Sons, Ltd. Companion website: www.ataglanceseries.com/TandO

Fractures around the knee
Distal femoral fractures

The distal femur comprises two condyles, which articulate with the tibia at the knee. A fracture may occur just above the level of the condyles, known as a supracondylar fracture, or extend in between the condyles, known as an intercondylar fracture. The mechanism is usually axial load combined with varus or valgus stress. In the elderly this may occur after a simple fall.

Undisplaced fractures may be treated in an above-knee cast, but these fractures usually displace due to the pull of the gastrocnemius muscle. Displaced fractures require surgery to restore alignment of the fragments and anatomical reduction of the joint surface. A plate and screws is the most commonly used fixation device. Retrograde intramedullary nailing may be used, although if the fracture is very low, it may prove difficult to secure the distal fragment with the locking screws in the nail. An alternative is to use a circular external fixator frame. This is a good option for highly comminuted fractures with extensive soft-tissue injury, but the frame is cumbersome, has to be in situ for several months and results in stiffness of the knee.

Patellar fractures

The patella is a sesamoid bone within the extensor mechanism of the knee. Superiorly is the quadriceps tendon, inferiorly the patellar tendon, and to either side a broad sheet of connective tissue known as the extensor retinaculum.

The patella may fracture in two ways: a direct fall onto a flexed knee resulting in a 'stellate' (star-shaped) comminuted fracture, or sudden contraction of the quadriceps muscle in an attempt to prevent a fall resulting in a transverse fracture across the patella. The fracture pattern is seen on lateral and AP knee X-rays.

Evaluation of the patient requires an assessment of the integrity of the extensor mechanism. This is achieved by asking the patient to perform a straight leg raise. With the leg straight, ask the patient to lift the heel off the bed. If the extensor retinaculum is intact, they will be able to lift the heel, and if the fracture fragments are undisplaced treatment is conservative in a cylinder cast. If the straight leg raise is negative, or the fracture is displaced, surgery is required.

Surgical treatment involves reducing the bone fragments anatomically in order to avoid arthritis beneath the patella. Fixation is usually achieved via a 'tension-band wiring'. This involves passing two parallel K-wires longitudinally across the patella, then bending a flexible wire over the top of the patella to the hold the fragments together. The torn extensor retinaculum is also repaired.

Tibial plateau fractures

The proximal tibia articulates with the femur at the knee. The tibial joint surface is relatively flat and comprises medial and lateral 'plateaux', separated by tibial spines representing the insertion of the cruciate ligaments.

Extreme valgus or varus force or axial loading across the knee may result in a tibial plateau fracture. Cruciate and meniscal injuries commonly coexist. Because the bone in this part of the tibia is relatively soft, the femoral condyles can either split the tibial plateau or cause depression of the joint line.

The fracture is classified according to whether lateral, medial or both plateaux are involved, and whether the bone is split, depressed or both. This is called the Schatzker classification. It is one of the few classifications that is useful to know:

Schatzker Classification

Type	Site	Configuration
I	Lateral	Split
II	Lateral	Depression
III	Lateral	Split and depression
IV	Medial	Any
V	Medial and lateral	Any
VI	Medial and lateral	Total separation of plateau from shaft

Treatment, as with all intra-articular fractures, is to restore the joint line anatomically. This is achieved with plate fixation. Areas of joint depression are elevated and it may be necessary to augment the fixation with bone graft or cement in order to prevent recurrent depression.

Tibial shaft fractures

The tibia may be fractured by a direct blow (transverse, butterfly or comminuted) or an indirect mechanism such as twisting (spiral). It is a common injury amongst footballers. The medial border of the tibia is just below the skin and open fractures are common. Compartment syndrome may result, especially following high-energy mechanisms where soft tissue may have been crushed. Severe unremitting pain should be considered compartment syndrome until proven otherwise.

Assess the neurovascular status, and assess skin integrity. X-rays should be carefully examined, looking for extension of the fracture into the knee or ankle joints.

Undisplaced fractures may be managed conservatively. Initially an above-knee cast is required. After 6–8 weeks this can be converted to a below-knee cast for a further 6–8 weeks. Regular monitoring with X-rays is essential to ensure alignment is maintained.

Displaced fractures require reduction and stabilisation. In some young patients a manipulation under anaesthetic and trial of plaster cast may be attempted, but the risk of late displacement is high.

Intramedullary nailing is commonly used. The nail is inserted proximally, through or adjacent to the patellar tendon. The nail allows the patient to be free of plaster, and depending on fracture configuration, weightbearing may be allowed immediately. Knee pain is common due to irritation of the patellar tendon.

Plate and screws may be used if the fracture extends into the knee or ankle. Wound breakdown may occur if the soft tissues are too swollen to allow a tension-free closure.

In open fractures, or in cases where the soft tissues are very swollen, an external fixator may be applied. This is usually a temporary solution as a precursor to nailing once the tissues allow, but may be definitive. The management of open fractures is discussed in more detail in Chapter 35.

43 Lower limb trauma 3

Figure 43.1   Weber classification
The level of the fibula fracture determines the classification. Weber A is never unstable, Weber B is sometimes unstable, Weber C is always unstable

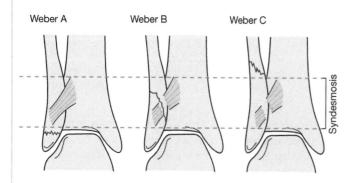

Weber A   Weber B   Weber C

Syndesmosis

Figure 43.2   Talar shift-in order to evaluate to talar shift obtain a true mortice view. The medial clear space should be equal to the superior clear space

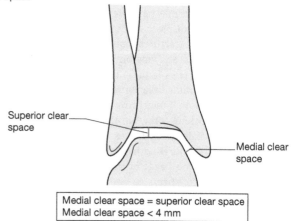

Superior clear space

Medial clear space

Medial clear space = superior clear space
Medial clear space < 4 mm

Figure 43.3   (a) Weber A fracture-the fibula fracture is below the level of the syndesmosis (b) Weber B fracture-the fracture is at the level of the syndesmosis but there is no talar shift. This can be managed conservatively (c) Weber B fracture with associated medial malleolus fracture, significant talar shift and dislocation of the ankle. This must be reduced as an emergency and definitively fixed once soft tissue swelling allows

(a)
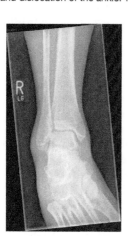

(b)
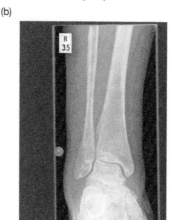

(c)
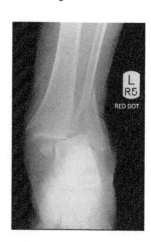

Figure 43.4   Injuries associated with fractures of the calcaneum

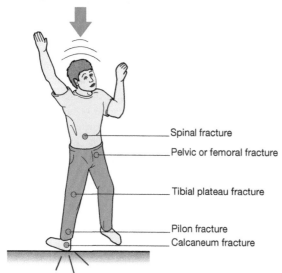

Spinal fracture
Pelvic or femoral fracture
Tibial plateau fracture
Pilon fracture
Calcaneum fracture

Figure 43.5   Lisfranc injury

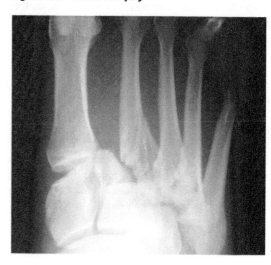

Trauma and Orthopaedics at a Glance, First Edition. Henry Willmott.
© 2016 John Wiley & Sons, Ltd. Published 2016 by John Wiley & Sons, Ltd. Companion website: www.ataglanceseries.com/TandO

Ankle
Relevant anatomy

The talus is a trapezoid-shaped bone that articulates with the tibia and fibula at the ankle. The tibia and fibula are bound together by the ligaments of the syndesmosis to form a mortise (a groove) in which the talus sits. The medial malleolus of the tibia stabilises the talus medially; the lateral malleolus of the fibula stabilises it laterally. Posteriorly, a lip of the tibial joint surface forms a posterior malleolus, which prevents the talus from subluxing backwards. Ligaments are also important stabilisers: medially the deltoid ligament and laterally the talofibular and calcaneofibular ligaments stabilise the joint.

Ankle fractures occur with twisting or axial loading mechanisms. Soft-tissue swelling is often severe. High elevation and ice are recommended. Examine carefully to determine areas of tenderness, paying particular attention to the medial side of the ankle in order to determine if the deltoid ligament has been torn.

Classification and treatment

Dislocation or gross displacement need urgent closed reduction to relieve pressure on the skin. Apply a below-knee backslab and obtain lateral and mortise views of the ankle.

Classification is helpful in determining treatment:

Weber classification

The level of the fibular fracture and the presence of talar shift determine treatment:

Weber A – fibular fracture below the level of the syndesmosis: The deltoid and syndesmotic ligaments are intact and the ankle is therefore stable. Treatment is in a below-knee cast or walking boot with weightbearing as tolerated.

Weber B – fibular fracture at the level of the syndesmosis: The critical question here is whether or not the ankle is stable. Instability is indicated by the presence of a medial malleolar fracture, the presence of a posterior malleolar fracture or the presence of talar shift. Talar shift is lateral subluxation of the talus due to loss of mortise stability – look for widening of the medial clear space. The gap should be the same all the way around the talus on the mortise-view X-ray. Any of these features on the X-ray indicate instability and are an indication for surgery, in the form of open reduction and internal fixation with plate and screws.

If no talar shift is seen, the ankle is probably stable and can be managed in a non-weightbearing below-knee cast for 6–8 weeks.

Weber C – fibular fracture above the level of the syndesmosis: These fractures are always unstable due to injury to the syndesmosis. The result is widening (diastasis) of the tibia and fibula. Treatment is open reduction and internal fixation of the fibula and stabilisation of the syndesmosis with screws or transosseous suture devices.

A special case is the **Maisonneuve fracture**. A twisting injury disrupts the syndesmosis and interosseous membrane between tibia and fibula. The fibula fractures high up around the knee and is therefore not seen on an ankle X-ray. If a patient has widening of the syndesmosis but no apparent fibular fracture, obtain full-length fibular X-rays and palpate the proximal fibula to try to find a fracture. Treatment is surgical stabilisation.

Pilon fractures

Severe axial loads may result in comminuted intra-articular fractures of the distal tibia. These are known as pilon fractures. Pilon is French for pestle (as in pestle and mortar), alluding to the impaction of the talus against the tibia.

The patient may have other injuries, so follow ATLS and examine carefully. Check neurovascular status and splint the limb in a backslab. Grossly displaced or dislocated ankles need urgent reduction. Often they are highly unstable and an external fixator may be required to maintain alignment.

Soft-tissue injury is extensive and may not develop fully for several days. High elevation and ice can help reduce swelling.

Definitive treatment is either plate fixation or a circular external fixator frame.

Calcaneum

Falling from a height onto the heel results in a calcaneal fracture. Associated with this injury are pilon fractures, tibial plateau fractures, pelvic fractures and spine fractures. All of these need to be actively looked for and excluded.

The joint between the calcaneum and the talus is known as the subtalar joint and it is often highly comminuted. Soft-tissue swelling is often severe. Admit for elevation and ice. Plaster casts are generally not required and can make things worse by exerting pressure on the skin.

Treatment is open reduction and internal fixation, attempting to realign the subtalar joint. The risk of arthritis and stiffness is high.

Lisfranc injury

The midfoot articulation is between the bases of the metatarsals distally and the cuneiforms and cuboid bones proximally. The joint is kept in alignment by the Lisfranc ligament. It runs between the base of the second metatarsal and the medial cuneiform.

Twisting or crush injuries to the foot may result in disruption of the Lisfranc ligament, often associated with fractures to one or more metatarsal bases.

Clinically the foot will be swollen with severe midfoot pain and bruising on the sole.

The injury is often difficult to see on X-ray and is frequently missed. The consequences of neglect are severe, with the development of midfoot arthritis, deformity and pain. If the diagnosis is unclear, request **weightbearing** AP and oblique views of the foot. Look for alignment of the medial border of the second metatarsal with the medial border of the middle cuneiform on the AP X-ray, and the medial border of the fourth metatarsal with the medial border of the lateral cuneiform on the lateral X-ray. If any doubt remains, a CT will confirm the diagnosis.

Treatment is surgical. Some surgeons prefer to use screws to reconstruct the midfoot and restore alignment. Others argue that the incidence of chronic pain is so high that a primary fusion of the midfoot is preferable. Controversy remains.

Summary of management of ankle fractures:

Weber A = conservative
Weber B with no talar shift = conservative
Weber B with talar shift = surgical
Weber C = surgical

(44) Proximal femoral fracture 1

Figure 44.1 Blood supply to femoral head
The main blood vessels are the ascending cervical branches which can be damaged if the femoral neck is fractured within the capsule

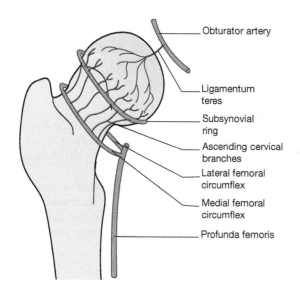

- Obturator artery
- Ligamentum teres
- Subsynovial ring
- Ascending cervical branches
- Lateral femoral circumflex
- Medial femoral circumflex
- Profunda femoris

Figure 44.2 Normal pelvis AP
Note intact Shenton's line and femoral neck trabeculae.

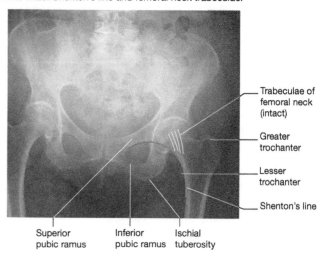

- Trabeculae of femoral neck (intact)
- Greater trochanter
- Lesser trochanter
- Shenton's line

Superior pubic ramus   Inferior pubic ramus   Ischial tuberosity

Figure 44.4 Normal lateral hip X-ray

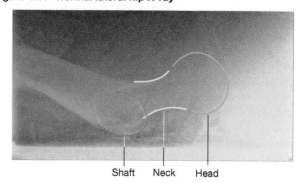

Shaft   Neck   Head

Figure 44.3 Classification of fractures by location-the integrity of the blood supply to the femoral head is determined by fracture location

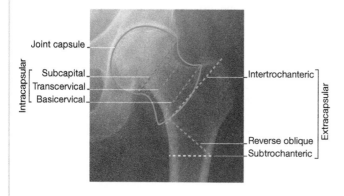

Joint capsule

Intracapsular
- Subcapital
- Transcervical
- Basicervical

Intertrochanteric

Extracapsular

- Reverse oblique
- Subtrochanteric

Figure 44.5 Clinical signs
If a patient has a displaced femoral neck fracture the leg will be shortened and externally rotated due to unopposed pull of muscle groups

Contusion   Pain NWB

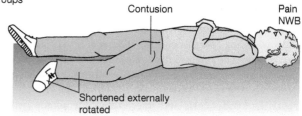

Shortened externally rotated

Trauma and Orthopaedics at a Glance, First Edition. Henry Willmott.
© 2016 John Wiley & Sons, Ltd. Published 2016 by John Wiley & Sons, Ltd. Companion website: www.ataglanceseries.com/TandO

Introduction

Fractures of the proximal femur, often referred to as 'hip fractures' or 'neck of femur fractures (NOF)', are common, accounting for a quarter of all fractures treated in UK hospitals. A proximal femoral fracture is often a marker of general frailty. In elderly patients they are associated with osteoporosis and may occur after a minor fall.

Outcomes after fractured NOF in the elderly

- 50% will not return to their pre-injury level of independence;
- 10% die within a month;
- 30% die within a year;
- common causes of death are pneumonia, pulmonary embolism (PE) and urosepsis.

In young patients, fractures around the hip are uncommon and are usually seen following major trauma. It is vital that these patients are managed according to the ATLS protocol and other life-threatening injuries excluded. This is discussed separately in Chapter 37.

Assessment of the elderly hip fracture patient

History

The fall is often fairly minor and from a standing height. Any elderly patient who complains of groin, buttock or thigh pain or is unable to mobilise after a minor fall should have X-rays.

The cause of the fall is often multifactorial, and cardiac, neurological and polypharmacy causes must be sought. Mental state examination should be conducted and recorded. A geriatrician's input is helpful.

Pathological fractures should be excluded, and any history of previous carcinoma (especially breast, prostate, lung or renal) should be taken seriously. The absence of a fall should also raise suspicion for pathological lesions. If there is any suggestion of a sclerotic or lytic lesion on the X-ray, obtain a full-length femoral X-ray to exclude any further lesions.

Examination

- **Look** – the patient will be in pain, unable to weightbear and with the leg shortened and externally rotated. This is due to unopposed pull of muscles around the hip. There may be bruising over the greater trochanter.
- **Feel** – the greater trochanteric region may be tender. Check the neurovascular status of the limb.
- **Move** – the patient will be unwilling to move the leg. Don't force them! Gentle internal and external rotation (by rolling the calf on the bed) will reproduce pain.
- **Other** – perform a top-to-toe examination. Ensure there is no head injury and that no other bones have been broken in the fall, especially shoulders and wrists.

Investigations

As with all fractures, two X-rays in perpendicular planes are essential. Request AP pelvis and lateral X-ray of the affected hip. It is wise to request a chest X-ray at the same time if it is likely the patient will require surgery.

Take blood as you would for any preoperative patient including group and save. Perform an ECG. Investigate appropriately if there is any suspicion of a medical cause for the fall. If you are questioning pathological fracture, a full-length femur X-ray, bone profile and relevant tumour markers should be sent. Remember to examine the prostate, breasts and abdomen.

Sometimes the diagnosis is unclear. The fracture may be incomplete, and a stoical patient may have attempted to mobilise causing the fracture fragments to become jammed together or impacted. Careful examination of the lateral X-ray may reveal the fracture – look for posterior displacement of the head relative to the neck, as if the 'ice cream has fallen off the cone'! Actively look for fracture of the pubic rami, which often presents in a similar fashion to neck of femur fracture. If doubt remains, MRI of the hips is the most sensitive and specific investigation. Some hospitals cannot provide this service, and will use CT instead. If doubt remains, a bone scan will show increased uptake at the fracture site.

45 Proximal femoral fracture 2

Figure 45.1   Is the fracture intra or extracapsular?

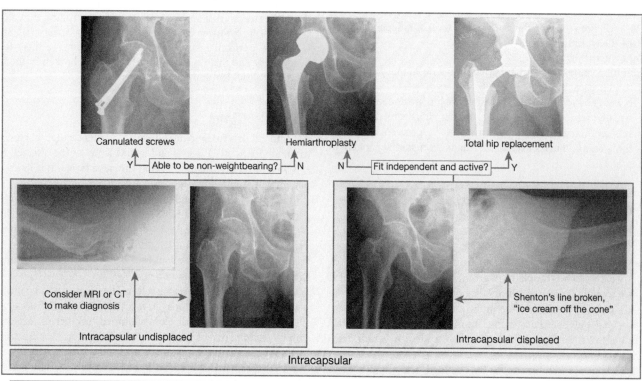

Cannulated screws   Hemiarthroplasty   Total hip replacement

Y — Able to be non-weightbearing? — N   N — Fit independent and active? — Y

Consider MRI or CT to make diagnosis   Shenton's line broken, "ice cream off the cone"

Intracapsular undisplaced   Intracapsular displaced

Intracapsular

Is the fracture intra or extracapsular?

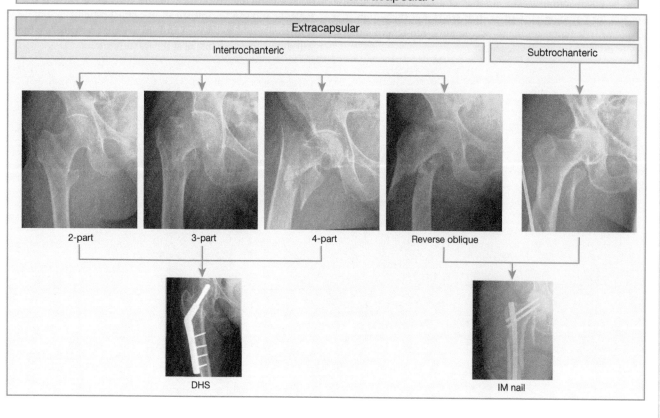

Extracapsular

Intertrochanteric   Subtrochanteric

2-part   3-part   4-part   Reverse oblique

DHS   IM nail

Trauma and Orthopaedics at a Glance, First Edition. Henry Willmott.
© 2016 John Wiley & Sons, Ltd. Published 2016 by John Wiley & Sons, Ltd. Companion website: www.ataglanceseries.com/TandO

Important anatomy
The blood supply to the femoral head

The blood supply to the femoral head originates from the profunda femoris artery, which gives off two branches, the medial and lateral femoral circumflex arteries. These loop around the base of the femoral neck to form the extracapsular ring. This gives off several small ascending cervical branches, which penetrate the capsule and run proximally within the joint, close to the femoral neck. When they reach the articular surface, they form the subsynovial intracapsular ring. This sends multiple tiny branches into the femoral head. The artery of the ligamentum teres is not clinically relevant in adults.

Clinical relevance of the blood supply

If the fracture is within the joint capsule (intracapsular), then the ascending cervical arteries may be disrupted, interrupting the blood supply to the femoral head. Fractures outside the capsule (extracapsular) are away from the ascending cervical branches and do not compromise the blood supply.

Classification and treatment
Intracapsular fractures

Intracapsular fractures risk damaging the blood supply to the femoral head. If the fracture is displaced, then the likelihood of subsequent avascular necrosis and non-union is high. It is an easy decision to replace the femoral head, usually with a hemiarthroplasty. In the fit, high-demand patient mobilising independently before the fall, the use of a total hip replacement is considered. This involves not only replacing the femoral head, but also relining the acetabulum with a cup. This is a bigger operation but removes the risk of acetabular erosion, a phenomenon seen in very active patients several years after a hemiarthroplasty.

Undisplaced intracapsular fractures are controversial. With no displacement, there is a possibility that the ascending cervical arteries are not torn and the head's blood supply is maintained. We therefore have the option of fixing the fracture with screws, rather than replacing the head. Screw fixation is a quicker and less invasive operation, but requires the patient to be non-weightbearing afterwards. Many elderly patients will be unable to comply with this. In addition, the risk of avascular necrosis still exists. If this occurs, it exposes the patient to further surgery. Many surgeons now argue that all intracapsular fractures, regardless of displacement, are best treated with a hemiarthroplasty.

Extracapsular fractures

Extracapsular fractures spare the femoral head blood supply. They can be divided into two main groups: intertrochanteric and subtrochanteric.

Intertrochanteric fractures run between the greater and lesser trochanters. The fracture can be simple, consisting of two large fragments of bone, or comminuted, consisting of three, four or more fragments of bone. Comminuted fractures are less stable. Most intertrochanteric fractures can be treated with a dynamic hip screw (DHS), which comprises a large screw in the femoral neck, coupled to a plate on the femoral shaft to which it is held with smaller screws. The pin can slide through the plate creating compression of the fracture when the patient bears weight.

Subtrochanteric fractures occur below the lesser trochanter. These fractures are highly unstable because of the unopposed pull of the various muscle groups around the hip. For this reason, the fractures tend to be fixed with an intramedullary (IM) nail, rather than a DHS. The nail is more difficult to position accurately than a DHS and complication rates are higher, but the fixation achieved is much more stable.

There is a variation of the intertrochanteric fracture known as **reverse oblique fracture** in which the fracture line extends obliquely from superomedial to inferolateral. A DHS, which allows sliding in an inferolateral direction, does not stabilise the fracture sufficiently and an intramedullary nail is required.

Postoperative treatment

These frail patients have undergone a big operation. Careful monitoring of observations and fluid balance is essential. A catheter is helpful, but should not routinely be left for more than 48 hours due to risk of urosepsis. Check haemoglobin and have a low threshold for transfusion. An X-ray is required following hemiarthroplasty or total hip replacement, but is not required for DHS or nails because X-rays are taken in theatre. All patients should have deep vein thrombosis (DVT) prophylaxis starting 12 hours post-op and continued until mobile.

Encourage the patient to mobilise early: the aim of surgery is to get the patient out of bed! Physiotherapy and occupational therapy are key. Patients should be fully weightbearing, unless otherwise stated in the notes. If a patient is slow to mobilise, arrange chest physio and prevent pressure sores.

Secondary falls prevention and anti-resorptive therapy for osteoporosis should be instigated for all patients. Discharge planning should start on day one. If the patient lived alone in a top-floor flat with no lift, will they realistically return there?

46 Cervical spine trauma

Figure 46.1

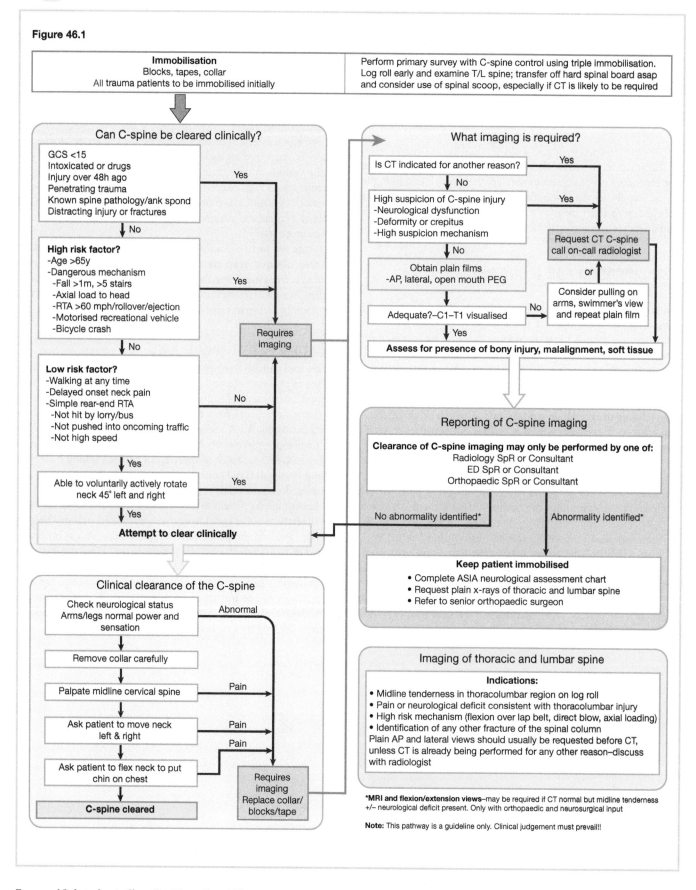

Assessing the cervical spine

Injuries to the cervical spine may occur after high-energy injuries such as motor vehicle accidents, or with relatively low-energy mechanisms such as sporting injuries. The combination of a stiff spine and osteoporosis in the elderly may result in spinal fracture following a fall from standing height.

All trauma patients should be assumed to have a cervical injury until proven otherwise. Spine protection is part of 'A' in the ATLS algorithm. Apply triple immobilisation – a rigid cervical collar, two sandbags and two lengths of tape across the stretcher.

Indications for cervical spine imaging

The Canadian C-spine rules determine which patients require X-rays. Patients over 65 years old, with a high risk mechanism, neurological symptoms or inability to move the neck freely require X-rays. See Figure 46.1 for details.

A lateral, AP and open-mouth view (to visualise the C2 peg) should be performed.

Interpretation of the X-ray

Adequacy – the whole cervical spine must be visible, from C1 down to the C7/T1 junction. Count the vertebrae to ensure this is the case. If C7/T1 is not visible, the shoulders may be in the way. Try repeating the lateral X-ray whilst gently pulling down on the patient's arms. Alternatively a swimmer's view adducts one arm as though the patient is doing front crawl. Failing this, request a CT.
- **Alignment** – trace four lines, looking for a step.
- **Bones** – trace the cortex of each bone, looking for a breach or step. Assess the facet joints for alignment.
- **Cartilage** – look at the disc spaces, are they equal?
- **Dens** – look at the dens (peg) of C2. Is it broken?
- **Everything else** – look for soft-tissue swelling. Soft-tissue depth greater than 6 mm at C2, or 22 mm at C6, may represent fracture haematoma.

If any doubt remains, get a CT.

Clinical examination of the C-spine

If imaging is normal, the spine must be cleared clinically by an experienced doctor.

First, perform a neurological examination of upper and lower limbs. With the patient lying still, gently remove the tape and sandbags. Open the collar and palpate in the midline for bony tenderness. If a tender spot is found, reassess the X-ray and consider the need for CT or MRI.

The patient must fulfil all of the following criteria before the collar can be removed:
- **No neurological deficit**;
- **No midline tenderness**;
- **No intoxication or reduced consciousness** (this may mean waiting until the patient is alert or sober);
- **No distracting injury**.

Remove the collar and ask the patient to slowly turn their head to either side and put their chin on their chest. If it is painful or neurological symptoms occur, stop and replace the collar.

Finish the examination by palpating for midline tenderness along the rest of the thoracolumbar spine.

Specific cervical spine injuries

C1 burst fracture

C1 is named the atlas, after the Greek mythological character who bore the world on his shoulders. C1 bears the weight of the head. Axial load applied to the top of the head, such as diving into a shallow swimming pool, can fracture C1 in a characteristic 'burst' pattern. The fracture is unstable and injury to the spinal cord at this level results in death. Treatment is surgical, either to fuse the skull to the spine, or to immobilise the cervical spine with a halo brace until healing occurs.

C2 peg fracture

The atlas rotates around a peg of bone arising from C2. The peg is also known as the dens. Hyperextension of the neck may result in fracture of the peg. It is a common injury in the elderly who fall from standing, hitting their chin on the floor and forcing the neck into extension. Most cases are treated with a collar for 8 weeks, but if the fracture is displaced or non-healing, screw fixation is possible.

Hangman's fracture

Combined distraction and extension, as occurs with hanging, may result in fracture of the C2 pedicles and disruption of the soft tissues between C2 and C3. Risk of spinal cord injury and quadriplegia is high. Treatment is surgical stabilisation.

Facet joint dislocation

The facet joints are obliquely orientated joints towards the posterior part of the vertebra. They allow movement to occur between adjacent vertebrae. Adjacent facet joints are normally congruent and aligned in parallel configuration. On a true lateral X-ray, the left and right facet joints directly overlie each other.

Distraction and flexion, as occurs with rapid deceleration, may result in dislocation of the facet joints. One side or both sides may be affected. The lateral X-ray demonstrates that one vertebra is subluxed anterior to the other, and congruence of the facets is lost, producing a double shadow.

The treatment is to reduce and stabilise the dislocation. The risk of spinal cord injury during the manoeuvre is high, as torn disc or ligamentous tissue may have been extruded into the spinal canal.

Body fracture

Hyperflexion combined with axial load may result in fractures of the anterior aspect of the vertebral body. This is also known as a teardrop fracture. If the force is sufficient, the posterior elements of the spine may be distracted, rendering the spine unstable. Surgical fixation is in the form of an anterior approach to the spine, combined with bone graft and fusion of adjacent vertebrae.

Clay shoveller's fracture

An avulsion of the tip of the C7 spinous process may occur due a sudden pull of the trapezius muscle. This historically happened when shovelling heavy unrelenting clay. The fracture is painful but stable and can be treated conservatively.

47 Thoracolumbar spine trauma

Figure 47.1   The three-column theory of spinal stability
Fractures involving one column are stable. Two or more column involvement implies instability

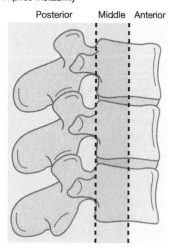

Figure 47.2   Wedge compression fracture
Only one column is involved so the fracture is stable. These are commonly seen in osteoporotic women falling from a standing height

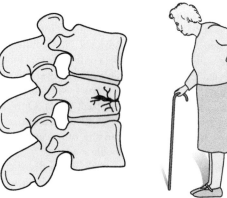

Figure 47.3   Burst fracture
Caused by extreme axial loading, such as a fall from a height. Two columns are involved. Fragments may be extruded into the spinal canal and result in neurological compromise. Surgical stabilisation may be required

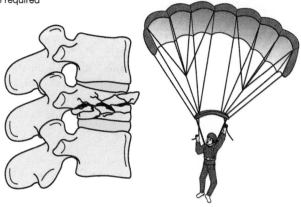

Figure 47.4   Chance fracture
Caused by extreme flexion and distraction, in car accident for example, three columns are involved. Displacement may transect the spinal cord

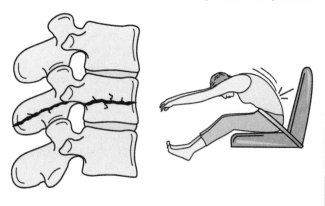

Trauma and Orthopaedics at a Glance, First Edition. Henry Willmott.
© 2016 John Wiley & Sons, Ltd. Published 2016 by John Wiley & Sons, Ltd. Companion website: www.ataglanceseries.com/TandO

Thoracolumbar fractures

Fractures of the thoracic or lumbar spine may occur as a result of high-energy mechanisms such as motor vehicle accidents and falls from a height. In the presence of osteoporosis or skeletal metastases, which weaken bone, fractures may occur after minimal trauma.

There are 12 thoracic and five lumbar vertebrae. The junction between these two segments is the most common site of fracture, because it is the transition zone between the relatively stiff thoracic spine and the much more flexible lumbar spine.

Assessment of suspected spinal fractures

If the mechanism is traumatic, manage the patient according to ATLS principles. Immobilise the patient on a flat bed, protecting the cervical spine with triple immobilisation precautions.

Perform and document a full neurological examination including a rectal examination. The American Spinal Injury Association (ASIA) publishes a helpful proforma to ensure the examination is complete. It is available at: http://www.asia-spinalinjury.org/elearning/ISNCSCI_Exam_Sheet_r4.pdf

Imaging

Obtain X-rays of the spine. If one area of the spine is fractured, there is a 5% risk of the patient having another spinal fracture at a different level. It is therefore advisable to X-ray the entire spine. Obtain AP and lateral views.

If the patient has multiple injuries, X-rays are inadequate, or a fracture is demonstrated, then CT is indicated.

Stability of spinal fractures

Unstable fractures may collapse, creating or worsening neurological injury and exacerbating deformity. Stability can be assessed using the 'three-column theory':

On the lateral X-ray, the spine is divided into three columns:
- The anterior column is the anterior half of the vertebral body, along with the anterior ligaments.
- The middle column is the posterior half of the vertebral body and the posterior ligaments.
- The posterior column is everything behind the vertebral body, including the pedicles, facet joints, laminae and spinous processes.

A fracture involving one column only is deemed stable, whereas a fracture involving two or more columns is unstable.

Specific types of spinal fracture

Wedge compression fracture

These fractures frequently affect elderly women who are osteoporotic. A simple fall from standing height onto the bottom is a classic mechanism. The presence of 'red flag' signs, absence of a fall, involvement of multiple vertebrae or past history of cancer should prompt consideration of bony metastases (see Chapter 27).

Only the anterior column is involved. The posterior border of the vertebral body is intact. This is a stable injury without risk of neurological injury because the spinal canal is not compromised.

Treatment is conservative with analgesia and gentle mobilisation. A corset-style brace may be used to help reduce pain. Surgery may be indicated if the fracture fails to heal (common in pathological fractures due to bony metastases) or if there is severe kyphosis.

One surgical option is vertebroplasty, whereby cement is injected into the vertebral body using a long needle inserted percutaneously under X-ray guidance.

Burst fracture

In contrast to a wedge fracture, a burst fracture involves two columns. The anterior and middle column are both fractured. The energy of the injury is therefore normally higher, and it occurs in younger patients who have fallen from a height.

Because the posterior wall of the vertebral body is involved, the spinal canal is compromised. There is a risk of neurological injury, either due to instability or by fragments of bone that have been pushed into the canal (known as 'retropulsion'). A CT is mandatory to evaluate this.

Treatment may be conservative in a brace. If there are neurological symptoms or significant deformity, surgery is indicated to stabilise the spine and decompress the cord.

Chance fracture

Extreme flexion combined with distraction results in a burst fracture to the anterior and middle columns, combined with distraction fracture to the posterior column. This can occur if a patient is wearing a lap-belt and has a head-on collision.

These fractures are highly unstable as all three columns are involved. Sometimes the posterior column injury may be purely ligamentous and only visible on MRI. Surgical stabilisation is necessary.

Transverse process fractures

Large muscles including the trapezius and psoas originate from the transverse processes. Avulsion fractures are fairly common when these muscles contract strongly in a side-impact collision, for example. Although the fractures are stable and heal without intervention, look carefully for other spinal or pelvic fractures that may coexist.

Spinal cord injury

Injury to the spinal cord may be made worse if the patient is not adequately resuscitated or the spinal column is not stabilised. The priority is to stick to the ATLS algorithm.

Cord injury may be complete or partial.

Complete cord injury is defined as no motor or sensory function below the level of injury. The priority in these cases is to prevent the injury from progressing and control pain by stabilising the spine with surgery, prevent complications and start rehabilitation.

The level of injury determines function:
- C1-2 – ventilator-dependent due to diaphragm paralysis;
- C6 – can flex arm to feed themselves;
- T2 – normal arm function;
- L1-5 – variable lower limb function, incontinent.

Spinal shock is a temporary shutdown of cord function due to recent trauma. During this period the injury level cannot be assessed. Spinal shock has finished when the bulbocavernosus reflex returns (anal contraction in response to tugging on the catheter).

Neurogenic shock is hypotension and bradycardia due to loss of sympathetic nerve function. It may be confused with hypovolaemia at first, but the key to diagnosis is the low pulse rate. Treat with vasopressor drugs.

Partial cord injury may take many forms, depending on which spinal tracts are affected. Recovery is sometimes possible.

48 Trauma in children 1

Figure 48.1 Fractures not involving the growth plate

(a) Torus fracture–the cortex has buckled but not broken. (b) Greenstick fracture–one cortex is broken, the opposite cortex is buckled. (c) Complete fracture–both cortices are broken and the fracture has displaced. The thick periosteum will be torn and may become interposed between the fracture fragments, making closed reduction difficult

(a)

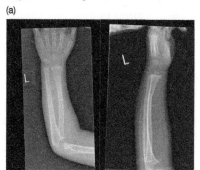

(b)

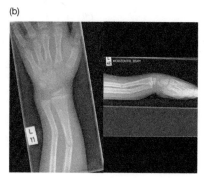

(c)

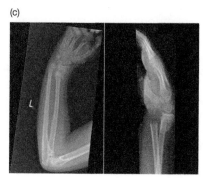

Figure 48.2 Anatomy of the growth plate

Mesenchymal stem cells at the bottom of the growth plate differentiate into chondrocytes which produce cartilage. The cartilage is ossified by osteoblasts at the top of the growth plate. Fractures may occur through this relatively weak area

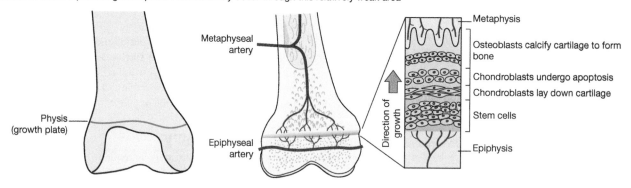

Figure 48.3 Salter-Harris classification of fractures involving the growth plate

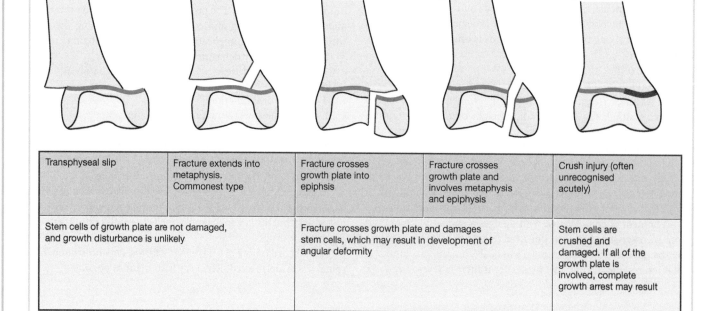

I	II	III	IV	V
Transphyseal slip	Fracture extends into metaphysis. Commonest type	Fracture crosses growth plate into epiphysis	Fracture crosses growth plate and involves metaphysis and epiphysis	Crush injury (often unrecognised acutely)
Stem cells of growth plate are not damaged, and growth disturbance is unlikely		Fracture crosses growth plate and damages stem cells, which may result in development of angular deformity		Stem cells are crushed and damaged. If all of the growth plate is involved, complete growth arrest may result

Trauma and Orthopaedics at a Glance, First Edition. Henry Willmott.
© 2016 John Wiley & Sons, Ltd. Published 2016 by John Wiley & Sons, Ltd. Companion website: www.ataglanceseries.com/TandO

Unique properties of children

There are some significant differences between children and adults.

Bone composition

At birth, the skeleton is largely cartilage. It becomes progressively more ossified as the child develops, but paediatric bones remain less brittle and more flexible than those of adults.

One clinical implication of this property is that injury to the chest or pelvis may result in significant visceral injury without fracture.

Fracture mechanisms

As a result of the different composition, the bone fractures in a different manner:

- **Plastic deformation** – minimal force may create a bend in a bone without cortical breach or fracture. Generally speaking such deformities remodel without the need for medical intervention.
- **Torus fractures** are also known as 'buckle fractures'. One side of the bone buckles on itself, whilst the contralateral side bends with plastic deformation. Torus fractures heal very quickly, typically within 2–3 weeks. They are stable and need only a removable splint for comfort.
- **Greenstick fractures** are a complete fracture on one side of the bone, combined with buckling on the other side.
- **Complete fractures** occur in a similar manner to adults – transverse with compression, butterfly or oblique with bending and spiral with twisting force.

Growth plates

The bones increase in length and width during development. Longitudinal growth occurs at the growth plates, also known as physes.

The growth plates are found at the ends of the bones. At one end of the growth plate are layers of stem cells that differentiate into chondrocytes to produce cartilage. At the opposite end of the growth plate, the chondrocytes undergo apoptosis and osteoblasts remodel the cartilage matrix into bone.

The growth plate is relatively weak compared to the bone. Fractures therefore commonly occur through the growth plate. These are known as 'physeal fractures'.

There are several distinct patterns of fracture, described by the Salter–Harris classification:

- **I:** Transphyseal fracture – the epiphysis slips off the metaphysis.
- **II:** Transphyseal fracture extending into the metaphysis of the bone. By far the commonest type.
- **III:** Transphyseal fracture extending into the epiphysis and the adjacent joint.
- **IV:** Fracture traversing the physis, starting in the metaphysis and extending into the epiphysis and joint.
- **V:** Crush injury to the physis. Rare.

Growth disturbance

Injury to the growth plate may result in damage to the layers of stem cells and subsequent disturbance of growth. In severe cases growth may be completely stopped on one half of the physis. If the unaffected half of the physis continues to grow, the result is progressive angular deformity.

Growth arrest is very uncommon in Salter–Harris (SH) types I and II. It is much more likely in III, IV and V, because the fracture line extends into the stem cell layer of the growth plate.

It is important to follow up children who have had a SH III, IV or V injury for some months or years after the fracture has healed in order to ensure that growth is not affected.

Thick periosteum

Longitudinal growth is produced by the physis, but growth in the transverse plane (increasing diameter) is provided by the periosteum. In adults the periosteum is a thin layer of tissue that sits on the surface of the bone. In children it is much thicker and stronger.

This can cause some problems when reducing displaced fractures. The thick periosteum can tear and a flap may become interposed in the fracture fragments. It is sometimes difficult to remove it from the fracture site without resorting to opening the fracture and removing it manually. One technique to try to flip the periosteum out of the fracture site is to exaggerate the deformity before applying longitudinal traction and corrective force.

Greater remodelling potential

Because children's bones are still growing, they have huge capacity to remodel after a fracture. This means that even quite large deformities can be accepted and as the bone continues to grow, it will correct the alignment itself.

Remodelling capacity is greatest in younger children, if the fracture site is close to the end of the bone and if the deformity is in the plane of movement of the adjacent joint.

Faster healing

Fractures heal much faster in children than in adults. In neonates, long bone fractures will heal in a matter of a couple of weeks.

Abundant callus is formed. Sometimes this can create a visible swelling at the fracture site, especially in skinny children. The parents should be reassured that this will remodel and decrease with time.

Non-accidental injury (NAI)

Child abuse may present with orthopaedic injuries and it is important to recognise the risk factors and features associated with NAI.

Injury inconsistent with the history:
- long bone fractures in a child not yet walking;
- spiral fractures suggesting twisting of the arm or leg.

Avoidance of healthcare providers:
- multiple visits to different hospitals in different areas;
- delayed presentation.

Physical examination findings:
- bruises, particularly in a grip or fingertip pattern;
- multiple fractures in different stages of healing.

Specific injuries:
- posterior rib fractures;
- skull fractures;
- petechial haemorrhages;
- torn frenulum.

Management

Report concerns to a senior and the named nurse for child protection. Admit the child to hospital until the situation is resolved.

49 Trauma in children 2

Figure 49.1 Ossification centres

There are six ossification centres around the elbow and they appear in a predictable sequential order

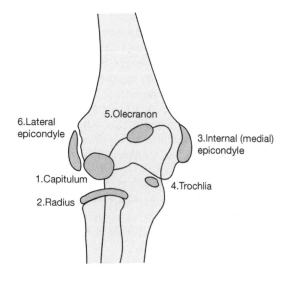

6. Lateral epicondyle
5. Olecranon
3. Internal (medial) epicondyle
1. Capitulum
4. Trochlia
2. Radius

Figure 49.2 AP elbow x-ray of a 4-year-old boy. The capitellum and radial head are the only visible ossification centres

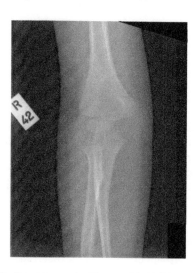

Figure 49.3 AP elbow x-ray of a 10-year-old girl. All the ossification centres are present, the lateral epicondyle is still very small

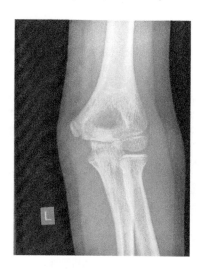

Figure 49.4 Normal elbow showing radiocapitellar and anterior humeral line

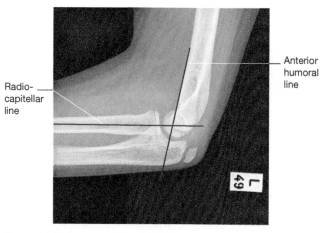

Anterior humeral line

Radio-capitellar line

Figure 49.5 Supracondylar fractures

(a) Gartland type 1: Undisplaced. Note the elevated fat-pads

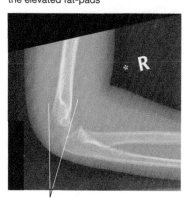

Elevated fat-pads

(b) Gartland type 2: Anterior cortex broken, posterior cortex hinged

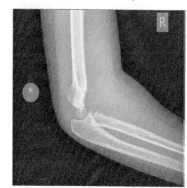

(c) Gartland type 3: Both anterior and posterior cortices are broken

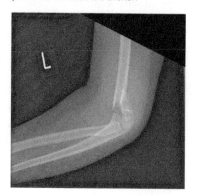

Trauma and Orthopaedics at a Glance, First Edition. Henry Willmott.
© 2016 John Wiley & Sons, Ltd. Published 2016 by John Wiley & Sons, Ltd. Companion website: www.ataglanceseries.com/TandO

Normal paediatric elbow anatomy
Ossification centres

The paediatric elbow is a common cause of confusion amongst junior doctors because it has six separate ossification centres, all of which appear at different ages. This makes interpretation of the X-ray difficult, as the small spots of bone may mimic fractures.

Knowledge of when the ossification centres are expected to appear is essential. The mnemonic **CRITOL** may be helpful:

	Girls	Boys
Capitellum	1	2
Radial head	3	4
Internal (medial) epicondyle	5	6
Trochlea	7	8
Olecranon	9	10
Lateral epicondyle	11	12

Remember, these are average ages. Individuals may vary, although the order remains the same.

X-ray interpretation

When looking at a child's elbow X-ray, ask yourself what ossification centres should be visible and check to see if they are there. If one is missing, is it fractured and displaced? If one is there which you think should not be there, is it a fracture fragment from elsewhere? If doubt still remains, consider X-raying the contralateral uninjured elbow for comparison.

The **fat pad**, or **'sail' sign**, is a sensitive way to evaluate the presence of a fracture. The elbow capsule has pads of fat in front and behind it. These appear grey on X-ray. If there is fluid within the elbow joint, the fat pads are pushed away from the bone and appear elevated from the humerus. In the context of trauma, fluid in the joint is probably blood, indicating that an intra-articular fracture is present.

There are two lines that help to assess alignment:
- The radial head can become dislocated in a Monteggia fracture or in isolation. The **radiocapitellar line** is an indication that the radial head is aligned with the capitellum. A line along the length of the radius should intersect the middle third of the capitellum on all views.
- The **anterior humeral line** is useful when assessing displacement in a supracondylar fracture. On the lateral X-ray a line along the anterior cortex of the humerus should intersect the anterior third of the capitellum.

Supracondylar fracture

This is the commonest paediatric elbow fracture and if displaced, carries a high risk of neurovascular injury. Peak incidence is between 4 and 8 years of age.

The mechanism is usually a fall onto an outstretched hand. Presentation is with severe pain and swelling and unwillingness to use the limb. Gross displacement may be visible as an S-shaped deformity.

Initial assessment

Perform a complete examination to exclude any other injuries, and then a careful examination of the neurovascular status.

The nerve most at risk is the anterior interosseous nerve (AIN), which may be injured in up to 10% of cases. The AIN is a branch of the median nerve, which innervates pronator quadratus, flexor pollicis longus (FPL) and flexor digitorum profundus (FDP) to the index and middle fingers. An easy way to test the latter two muscles is to ask the child to make an 'OK' sign. If the AIN is damaged, the child will unable to flex the index finger distal interphalangeal joint (DIPJ) and thumb interphalangeal joint (IPJ) to make a perfect circle.

The remaining nerves should also be checked, which is not easy in a screaming child! Try asking the child to play 'paper, scissor, stone'. The flat 'paper' hand tests the radial nerve and posterior interosseous nerve (PIN); the clenched 'stone' tests the median nerve and anterior interosseous nerve (AIN); the 'scissor' movement tests the ulnar nerve.

True **vascular injury** is present in around 1% of cases, although arterial spasm is much more common. Check the radial pulse and the capillary refill in the fingers. A pulseless limb is an emergency and requires urgent intervention.

X-rays

Obtain AP and lateral elbow X-rays. The amount of displacement determines management and is classified by the Gartland system:
- Gartland 1: non-displaced. Fat pads may be the only sign.
- Garland 2: displaced with intact posterior cortex.
- Gartland 3: completely displaced.

Treatment

- Gartland 1 fractures may be managed in an above-elbow cast with the elbow flexed to around 90° for 3–4 weeks.
- Gartland 2 fractures require reduction under anaesthesia. If the fracture is felt to be unstable, K-wires may be used to stabilise the fracture.
- Gartland 3 fractures need reduction and pinning in theatre. Sometimes it is very hard to achieve and maintain reduction percutaneously and the elbow will have to be opened. There is some controversy about the urgency of surgery in these cases. If there is neurovascular compromise, many surgeons will want to operate as soon as possible – even in the middle of the night. Others feel it can wait until morning, but let your senior make that decision and notify them immediately!

Medial epicondyle fracture

The medial epicondyle may be pulled off by the strong flexor muscles that originate here. Up to 50% of cases are associated with an elbow dislocation. There is a danger that the medial epicondyle may become trapped within the joint as the elbow reduces. This is difficult to see, but the clue is a 'missing' medial epicondyle on the X-ray with medial tenderness and swelling. Remember CRITOL – if the 'I' is missing, when it should be there, look carefully in the joint and X-ray the opposite elbow for comparison if you are unclear.

Minimally displaced medial epicondyle fractures are treated conservatively in an above-elbow cast for 3–4 weeks. If the fragment is incarcerated in the joint, surgery is required.

Lateral condyle fracture

The lateral condyle may be pushed off by valgus force across the elbow, or pulled off by varus force. It is quite a common injury.

Management is determined by the amount of displacement. Less than 2 mm displacement may be managed conservatively in a cast. More than 2 mm requires reduction and fixation with K-wires.

Failure to recognise or treat the injury appropriately may result in progressive valgus deformity at the elbow.

50 Compartment syndrome

Figure 50.1 Anatomy of myofascial compartments

The arm has two compartments, the forearm has four. The thigh has three compartments, the leg has four

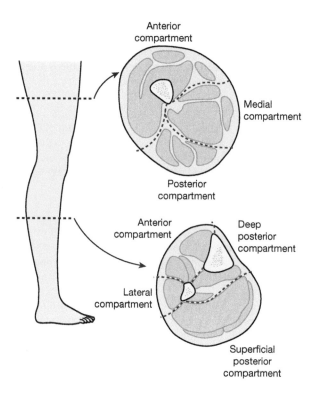

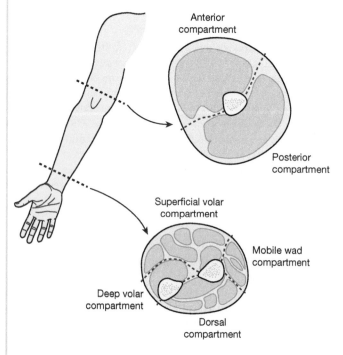

Figure 50.2 Symptoms of compartment syndrome

Pain out of proportion to injury. Passive stretching of affected muscles increases pain: Dorsiflexion of the great toe and ankle stretches muscles in the posterior compartments, plantar flexion stretches muscles in the anterior compartment. Tense compartments, loss of sensation, loss of pulses and pallor are late, insensitive signs and should not be relied upon

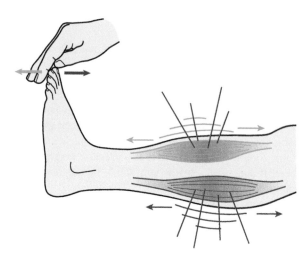

Figure 50.3 Treatment is by fasciotomy

Every compartment in the limb must be released. In the lower leg this is achieved via two long incisions, one medial the other lateral. The fascia is split and left open until swelling in the muscles has resolved

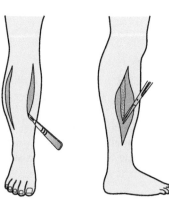

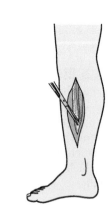

Trauma and Orthopaedics at a Glance, First Edition. Henry Willmott.
© 2016 John Wiley & Sons, Ltd. Published 2016 by John Wiley & Sons, Ltd. Companion website: www.ataglanceseries.com/TandO

Definition

Compartment syndrome is defined as increased pressure within a myofascial compartment that exceeds capillary perfusion pressure resulting in muscle ischaemia.

In plain English, the muscles of the limbs are contained within fascial compartments. The fascia is tough fibrous tissue that cannot expand. An increase in volume of the contents of the compartment increases the pressure.

Small variations in pressure are quite normal: sitting on a limb for a few minutes increases the pressure; exercise results in vasodilation in the muscle belly resulting in increased pressure; contraction of a muscle increases the pressure.

However, if the pressure increases to an extent that is greater than the perfusion pressure, blood will be unable to get into the compartment. The result is ischaemia. If ischaemia is ongoing, muscle necrosis results.

Aetiology

Compartment syndrome can occur due to:
- **Fractures** – any fracture may result in compartment syndrome, although it is more common with high-energy comminuted fractures.
- **Crush injuries** – either lying on the floor for a long period after a fall, or a more acute crush with a heavy weight damages the muscle resulting in significant swelling. Rhabdomyolysis may coexist so measure creatinine kinase and ensure the patient is well hydrated to prevent kidney injury.
- **Soft-tissue injury or contusions** – muscle swelling increases compartment pressure.
- **Tight casts or dressings** – this is the most common reversible cause of compartment syndrome. An injured limb will swell for up to 48 hours. Tight casts or dressings restrict vascular outflow and result in compartment syndrome. Although a backslab should allow some expansion, it may be insufficient. Increasing pain should prompt release of all dressings, all the way down to skin.
- **Extravasation of IV infusion** – infusion of fluid via a malpositioned IV cannula may result in compartment syndrome, especially in the hand where muscle compartments are small.
- **Burns**, especially electrical – burns may cause compartment syndrome in two ways: burnt skin contracts and becomes tight, squeezing muscle compartments; electrical burns pass through muscle en route to earth, resulting in muscle swelling.
- **Post-ischaemic swelling** – if a limb is revascularised, significant vasodilation and hyperaemia result in an attempt to flush out metabolic waste. This may result in muscle swelling and compartment syndrome.
- **Bleeding disorders or intramuscular haematoma** – patients with coagulopathies or on warfarin may develop a spontaneous intramuscular haematoma, which can be large enough to cause compartment syndrome. Treatment should include reversal of warfarin if necessary.

Symptoms and signs

Pain, pain, pain! The most sensitive symptom is pain. Muscle ischaemia results in pain that is out of proportion to the injury. The pain is exacerbated by stretching the affected muscles. This is called **passive stretch pain**: moving the big toe upwards stretches flexor hallucis longus (FHL) in the deep flexor compartment of the calf; moving the big toe downwards stretches extensor hallucis longus (EHL) in the anterior compartment.

As ischaemia worsens, sensory nerves are affected. The patient complains of pins and needles, and in advanced stages of compartment syndrome, loss of sensation.

Loss of peripheral pulses is an extremely late sign.

Palpating compartments to see if they are swollen or 'tight' has poor sensitivity.

Measuring compartment pressure

Unconscious patients will be unable to complain of pain. Sometimes ITU doctors or anaesthetists may note persistent tachycardia and hypertension suggestive of a pain response.

The pressure within the compartments may be measured in A&E or on the ward using a needle attached to a pressure transducer. If a dedicated machine is not available, an arterial line transducer can be set up to perform this function. Compartment pressures within 30 mmHg of the diastolic blood pressure represent compartment syndrome. This technique is inaccurate, however, and if compartment syndrome is a concern, it is safest to proceed with surgical decompression.

Treatment

Fasciotomy is the treatment. The muscle compartments are decompressed via long incisions along the limb, opening the skin, fat and fascia. If pressure is elevated, the muscle bulges out through the incisions. The wounds are not closed at the initial operation. Instead, the swelling is allowed to settle and the patient is returned to theatre after 48–72 hours for a second look. If the skin can be closed without tension this is done. If not, skin grafts may be required.

Neglected compartment syndrome

If compartment syndrome is not recognised and goes untreated, the result is muscle necrosis. In the acute phase this may result in renal failure due to rhabdomyolysis. Long-term, the dead muscle becomes scarred and contracted. This is known as **Volkmann's ischaemic contracture**. The clinical manifestations depend on which compartments are affected but include clawing of the toes, foot drop, equinus contracture, stiffness of the knee or clawing of the hand. The condition is irreversible and very disabling.

Chronic exertional compartment syndrome

Athletes sometimes complain of severe pain in the calves after running long distances or 'shin splints'. This is due to a chronic, low-grade compartment syndrome. As they exercise, the muscles of the leg swell and if the fascia of the calf is too tight blood flow is restricted, resulting in pain. Symptoms settle quickly with rest.

Treatment is release of the affected compartments via elective fasciotomy.

51 Non-union and malunion

Figure 51.1 Factors affecting bone healing
Nutrition, blood supply to the fracture fragments, and presence of bone-forming cells are essential, Smoking, malnutrition (especially lack of calcium and vitamin D), a high-energy mechanism or comminuted fracture pattern and instability are risks for nonunion

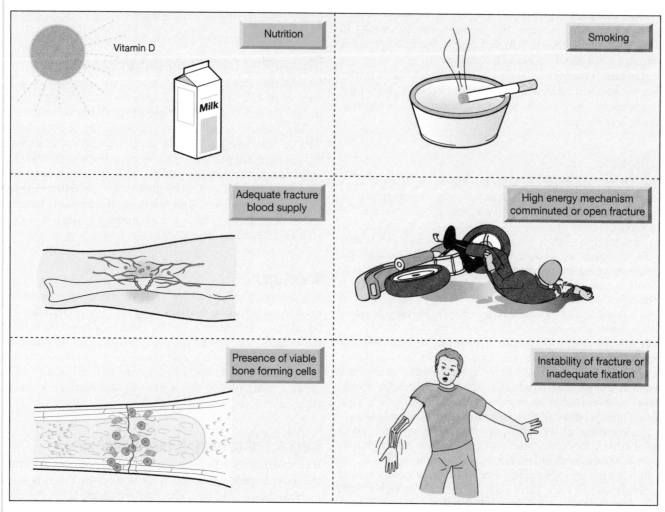

Nutrition

Vitamin D

Milk

Smoking

Adequate fracture
blood supply

High energy mechanism
comminuted or open fracture

Presence of viable
bone forming cells

Instability of fracture or
inadequate fixation

Figure 51.2 Types on nonunion
Hypertrophic nonunion is a result of inadequate stability. Atrophic nonunion is a result of inadequate biological response–lack of blood supply to fracture fragments, malnutrition or lack of bone-forming cells

Figure 51.3 Types of malunion

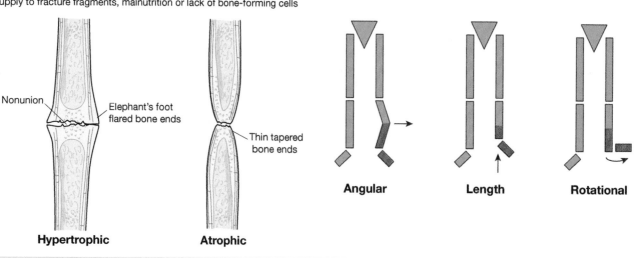

Nonunion

Elephant's foot
flared bone ends

Thin tapered
bone ends

Hypertrophic

Atrophic

Angular

Length

Rotational

Trauma and Orthopaedics at a Glance, First Edition. Henry Willmott.
© 2016 John Wiley & Sons, Ltd. Published 2016 by John Wiley & Sons, Ltd. Companion website: www.ataglanceseries.com/TandO

Definitions

Delayed union: A delayed union is when a fracture does not heal within the expected time.

Non-union: A non-union is defined as any fracture that has failed to heal within 9 months.

Fracture healing

There are two prerequisites for a fracture to heal:

Adequate biology – an inadequate healing response results in failure of callus formation. This is called *atrophic non-union*. The bone ends have a thin, tapered appearance with no callus visible.

Adequate stability – if a fracture is not stabilised during the healing process, despite the formation of callus, the fracture will not heal. The result is a *hypertrophic non-union*. The radiographic appearance is of abundant callus, which has been described as resembling an elephant's foot.

Causative factors

The causes of non-union may be thought of as internal or external:

Internal factors

- **Blood supply** – the fracture site needs an adequate blood supply to provide nutrients for the healing to occur. If the bones have been stripped of their periosteum, either by a violent mechanism of injury or an over-exuberant surgeon, the blood supply to the bone is compromised and atrophic non-union may result. Patients with diabetes and peripheral vascular disease have poor circulation and fractures take longer to heal in these individuals.
- **Malnutrition** – healing a fracture requires significant amounts of nutrients. Inadequate calorific intake, lack of calcium or vitamin D can result in delayed healing. The triad of anorexia, low bone density and amenorrhoea is known as the female athletic triad and puts the patient at risk of stress fractures and non-unions.

External factors

- **Smoking** – a very common cause of delayed or non-union, smoking acts in several ways to slow the bone healing process: nicotine directly inhibits osteoblasts, and the combination of carbon monoxide inhalation and vasoconstriction reduces oxygen delivery to the tissues.
- **Instability** – you will recall from Chapter 36 that bone heals either by primary or secondary means. Secondary healing occurs via callus formation. Callus formation is stimulated by *micromovement* at the fracture site. However, too much movement results in the production of granulation tissue, resulting in non-union. Primary healing requires absolute stability and direct apposition of the bone ends. If a fracture is rigidly plated but the bone ends are not reduced, and remain separated by a gap, there is no micromovement to stimulate callus formation, but the gap does not allow primary bone healing and non-union will result.

Treating delayed or non-union

Assess stability and reduction

If the fracture is too mobile, callus cannot bridge the fracture site. The treatment is to improve stability. This may entail making the patient non-weightbearing, applying a more stable cast or stabilising the fracture via surgical means such as a plate or intramedullary nail. Conversely, a fracture that has been plated but inadequately reduced may have separation of the bone ends and require revision surgery.

Improve biological activity

In order for healing to occur, the fracture needs three things:

1 cells to make bone;
2 signalling molecules to tell the cells to make bone;
3 a scaffold to lay bone upon.

In normal circumstances, these criteria are met by the fracture haematoma. In the context of a non-union, several months after the initial injury, the haematoma will no longer be present. There are two ways in which the three essential healing elements can be provided:

- **Creation of a new fracture haematoma** – surgically 'freshing up' the bone ends using drills or saws will result in bleeding. The new haematoma will aid bone healing.
- **Application of bone graft** – taking bone from elsewhere in the body provides fresh bone cells, signalling molecules and a scaffold to help the fracture ends heal. Commercially available products include synthesised signalling molecules in a putty or paste to stimulate the patient's own bone cells to produce callus.

Adjuncts to aid fracture healing

Various external stimuli have been shown to improve bone healing. Two examples are ultrasound and electric current applied across the fracture site. In theory, these stimuli increase activation of osteoblasts.

Malunion

If a fracture heals in the wrong position, this is known as a malunion. Malunions are described in terms of alignment, rotation and shortening. Malunion may be well tolerated, especially when close to a joint and in the same plane as the joint movement. Although the malunion may change the arc of movement of the joint, function is often not affected.

Malunions with significant angulation or rotation may affect function. The deformity can be corrected; correction techniques include:

- **Orthoses**: a brace to limit movement and restore stability to a joint is an option if surgery is to be avoided.
- **Osteotomy**: cutting or 're-breaking' a bone. Once the bone is cut, it can be repositioned using a plate or external fixator frame. Often bone graft is used to encourage the osteotomy to heal.
- **Hemiepiphysiodesis**: in children whose physes are still growing, angular deformities can be corrected by selectively fusing half of the growth plate. The unfused half of the growth plate continues to grow, resulting in the bone remodelling in the required direction. This requires careful planning and is only useful in children with a number of years' growth remaining.

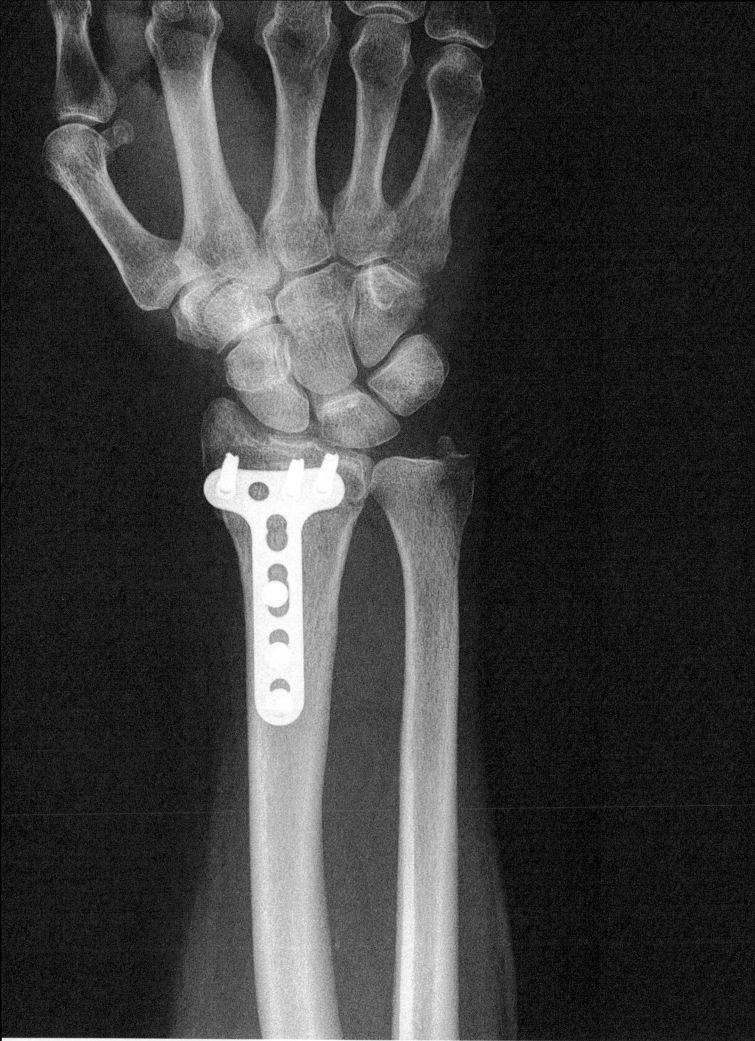

Working as a junior doctor in orthopaedics

Part 5

Chapters

Visit the companion website at **www.ataglanceseries.com/TandO** to test yourself on these topics.

Being an orthopaedic F2

Figure 52.1

Overview

For many Foundation Doctors, their orthopaedic placement is a daunting prospect. It is easy to understand why: many medical schools do not teach much orthopaedics, and what they do teach is often bundled together with rheumatology, a very different specialty. There are a number of aspects of orthopaedics that are alien to the other specialties, including metal implants, screws, nails, power tools, etc. Finally the structure of the job is very different, and you may find yourself working much more independently than in previous placements.

New doctors may therefore feel inadequately equipped for the job. There is fear of the unknown. Hopefully this book will go some way to addressing that.

Whilst sitting in the mess, I have overheard junior doctors complaining that they feel that orthopaedics is not relevant to them, as they want to be a GP or a physician. But what other job will allow you to take as much control over managing medical problems on the ward as you wish? Besides, even if you end up being a public health doctor, your friends will still expect you to know what to do if someone breaks a bone.

Trauma and Orthopaedics at a Glance, First Edition. Henry Willmott.
© 2016 John Wiley & Sons, Ltd. Published 2016 by John Wiley & Sons, Ltd. Companion website: www.ataglanceseries.com/TandO

Your responsibilities

There are three main aspects to your job as an orthopaedic doctor:

1. Ward work

The precise structure of the firm will vary between hospitals, but you will be responsible for the care of the inpatients under one or more consultants. You must see **all** of your patients **every** day and write in their notes. The timetable of ward rounds varies, but commonly the registrar will do a round twice a week or more, whereas consultants tend to do a round once a week. Ask them what their preferences are. On the days when there is no formal ward round, you are in charge! This may be the first time in your career when you are in this situation. It might be tempting to cut corners, but you have a duty of care to your patients. Go and see them, talk to them, elicit their concerns and be a good doctor.

Efficiency is essential. Make a computerised list and update it throughout the day. It is easiest to have this on a shared network drive so everyone in the team can access it. A really good F2 will present his or her registrar and consultant with an up-to-date list every morning. By keeping it comprehensive and accurate, weekend handover lists can easily be created.

When patients are discharged, do not delete them from the list. Instead, copy the relevant text to a separate page or file. This makes monthly morbidity and mortality meetings much easier to organise.

2. On call

Although you will be busy, seeing and treating new patients is a really fun part of the job. The key to surviving on calls is organisation.

When you are on call, carry the following items:

- Pen and paper – keep a list of *every* phone call and referral.
- Permanent marker pen – for marking limbs.
- Stethoscope – the registrar and consultant won't have one!
- A decent pair of blunt-tipped scissors for cutting dressings.
- Clerking proformas.
- Consent forms – although you will not take consent, it helps the registrar if you've got a form with stickers applied!
- Mobile phone of registrar – especially at night.

Being on call entails considerable responsibility. In most hospitals, you will be the first port of call for A&E and GPs. Always be polite to people on the phone, even if the referral is inappropriate. Play safe and accept all referrals. Until you have seen and examined the patient yourself, you cannot make a judgement. A favourite of A&E, especially nurse practitioners, is to ask for you to 'have a quick look at an X-ray'. You are not a radiologist. Go and examine the patient.

If in doubt, ask for help.

3. Theatre and clinic

These are not optional! During your 4 months in orthopaedics, you must get to theatre and clinic. By organising your time efficiently and sharing ward cover with your colleagues, you will be able to find time.

If you are keen, turn up and show interest, you will be allowed to scrub in and get involved. Most F2s will be allowed to close wounds and if you come to theatre regularly you will be allowed to do more.

Referring up the chain

If in doubt, ask for advice! Your registrar will not mind you calling him or her provided you do it in the right way. Let me give you an example:

Hi, Dave, its Kevin the on call orthopaedic SHO today. Sorry to bother you but I want some advice about a new referral I've just seen in A&E. I have an elderly lady with a distal radius fracture. The patient is an otherwise fit and well independent 80-year-old right-handed lady who had a mechanical fall from standing height this morning, sustaining a fracture of her left distal radius. It's an isolated injury, closed and neurovascularly intact. The fracture is dorsally angulated with some comminution and it extends intra-articularly. I've put in a haematoma block and tried to manipulate it and applied a below-elbow backslab. Although the angulation has improved somewhat, it's still shortened and I think it might need surgery. Would you mind having a look please?

When you make the call:

- Remind the registrar who you are (especially at the start of the job or at night when s/he's half asleep!).
- Say what you want – verbal advice or physical assistance.
- One sentence prologue – e.g. 'I have a man with an open tibial fracture.'
- Patient demographics and *relevant* past medical history (PMH).
- Hand dominance in upper limb injuries.
- Mechanism of injury.
- Isolated (ATLS), N/V intact, closed?
- X-ray description (PARTS acronym).
- Intervention so far.
- What you think might need to be done.
- Repeat what you want.

Presenting in trauma meetings

Although this may seem daunting, if you stick to a structure you won't go wrong. It is very similar to making a referral on the telephone. Remember that no one expects you to know exactly what to do with every patient.

- *This is...* name, age, sex, occupation, hand dominance, concise past medical history and AMTS if relevant.
- Mechanism of injury.
- Injuries sustained – if multiple injuries, run through the ATLS ABCDE then top-to-toe findings in secondary survey.
- Neurovascular status and open/closed.
- *The X-ray shows...* see Chapter 5.
- What has been done so far.
- *In summary...* don't repeat the whole thing, but try to condense it down to one or two sentences.
- *My plan with this patient is...* this is where you can shine, but even if you're not sure, have a go – you probably do know the answer!

A few final tips

- Document everything. Everything!
- Ask for help early – get the registrar's mobile number.
- Remember DVT prophylaxis.
- Don't forget analgesia.
- Put yourself in the patient's shoes – what would you want? Keep patients and families informed about treatment plans.
- Never lie – if you haven't done something or don't know the answer, say so!

53 Assessment of patients

Figure 53.1 Assessment proforma for new patients

Patient details

Adressograph label

Clerking by:
Date:...../...../20...   Time: ..... : .....
Consultant:
Registrar:
Referral from: A&E/#clinic/ward

Presenting complaint:

History of presenting complaint:

Time of injury: ..... : .....   Mechanism: Last ate and drank: ..... : .....
Isolated injury Y/N
If N, ATLS primary survey done?....................
Secondary survey done?...........................   Other injuries ....

Treatment so far:

☐ Analgesia   ☐ Tetanus
☐ Reduction   ☐ Antibiotics
☐ Backslab   ☐ Repeat x-ray

Past medical history:

Drug history:

Allergies: ☐ Warfarin   ☐ Asprin   ☐ Clopidogrel

Social circumstances:
Alone/carer at home   Job
Stairs   Right/Left handed
Orthoses   Smoker: Y/N
Exercise tolerance

Examination findings:

ATLS:	Abdo	X-ray findings:
☐ A		☐ Adequate?
☐ B		☐ AP/Lat?
☐ C		
☐ D		
☐ E		

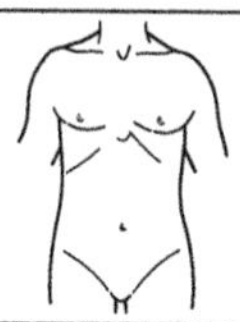

Chest	Pulses	Blood results:
		Hb........... INR.............
		Crt........... Other:
		Na........... G&S/X-match......Units
		K.............

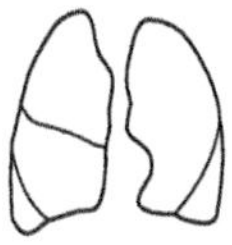

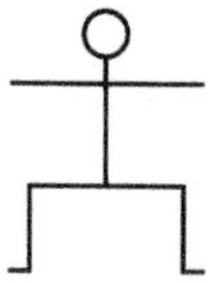

Neurology (use ASIA score for spinal injury)
          R   L
UL   Power   ☐   ☐
     Sens   ☐   ☐
LL   Power   ☐   ☐
     Sens   ☐   ☐

Injured limb examination:
Pulses.......................   Cap refill................
Sensation..................   Wounds.................
Deformity..................

Diagnosis:

Plan
Reduce? A&E/theatre?   ☐ Post MUA or POP x-ray result:
Plaster or splint?
Conservative-safe for d/c
Admit: Ward......   ☐ Follow-up arranged:
Surgery-Inform Spr, anaesthetics, theatre
        Consent:
        Mark:

Signed:
Date and time:
Bleep number:

Trauma and Orthopaedics at a Glance, First Edition. Henry Willmott.
© 2016 John Wiley & Sons, Ltd. Published 2016 by John Wiley & Sons, Ltd. Companion website: www.ataglanceseries.com/TandO

Emergency admissions from clinic or A&E

As an orthopaedic Foundation Doctor, you will frequently be asked to arrange admission of trauma patients, either in A&E or in fracture clinics. The most common reason for admitting a patient is for surgery, and your clerking should be focused in this respect.

Stick to the time-honoured format:

• Presenting complaint – ask specifically about the mechanism of injury, associated injuries, loss of consciousness, neck or back pain, etc.

• Past medical history – this may be extensive, but try to focus on the aspects relevant to surgery, especially cardiac or pulmonary disease, which may complicate anaesthesia.

• Drug history – ask specifically about aspirin, clopidogrel or warfarin, which may increase bleeding after surgery.

• Allergies – antibiotics are particularly common. Ask also about shellfish, as this may coexist with intolerance of iodine, which is commonly used to clean the skin in theatre.

• Social history – always ask about the patient's living arrangements as this will influence discharge options.

• Examination – always examine the heart and lungs, as it is unlikely that the orthopaedic registrar or consultant will do this! Document the neurovascular status of the injured limb, and in the context of spinal injury, perform and document a full neurological examination using the ASIA chart to help you.

• Investigations – your orthopaedic seniors will guide you as to what preoperative radiographic investigations are required. If the patient is being admitted for surgery, it is always sensible to request a chest X-ray in patients over 65 years old or with positive examination findings. Young patients having minor surgery do not normally require blood tests. Blood should be taken for FBC and U&E as a baseline in older patients. Add INR or coagulation profile if they are taking warfarin. If infection is suspected, measure CRP or ESR. If the patient is having major surgery, such as fixation of a long bone, a fracture around a major joint or in the context of significant trauma, take blood for group and save. If significant bleeding is anticipated, arrange cross-matching according to the hospital policy.

Specific issues

Pathological fractures

The commonest cause of a pathological fracture is metastases from a primary tumour elsewhere. In many cases the primary is known, which makes subsequent treatment of the fracture much easier. Sometimes a patient will present with a pathological fracture without a prior diagnosis of cancer. In these cases it is important to find the primary source.

The history may be helpful. Ask about weight loss, pain, rectal bleeding, haemoptysis, history of smoking or previous cancers.

Perform a careful abdominal and rectal examination. Examine the chest and the breasts in a female. Palpate the prostate in men.

A chest X-ray is mandatory. A CT of the chest, abdomen and pelvis will identify any other metastases and may identify the primary.

Systemic manifestations of tumour metastasis may include anaemia due to gastric blood loss, coagulopathy due to liver involvement, hyponatraemia due to syndrome of inappropriate antidiuretic hormone (SIADH) secretion, and hypercalcaemia or elevated ALP due to bone involvement. Send FBC, U&E, bone profile, clotting screen and LFTs.

Specific tumour markers should not be used for screening, but can be helpful in assessing progression of known tumours.

The oncology team will be able to offer further advice and will coordinate ongoing management. If they already know the patient, inform them of his/her admission.

Reversal of warfarin

Warfarin acts by inhibiting the production of vitamin K-dependent clotting factors. Its effects last for around 5 days until it has been metabolised and the clotting factors replenished by the liver. For elective operations, warfarin is stopped a week before surgery. In the emergency context, this will not be possible.

In the first instance, check the INR. Many surgeons will be happy to operate with an INR of less than 1.5. Most anaesthetists may be reluctant to perform a spinal anaesthetic unless the INR is less than 1.3. Check with your consultant.

If the patient is not actively bleeding and surgery can wait for 12–24 hours, the easiest way to reverse the warfarin is to administer vitamin K. In the first instance give 1 mg IV. Check the INR 8–12 hours later. If is still high, repeat the dose.

If the patient is actively bleeding or surgery must be performed immediately, there are two options. Fresh frozen plasma (FFP) takes around an hour to be matched and defrosted. Its effects last around 6 hours, so it should be given immediately before the start of surgery. The alternative to FFP is prothrombin complex concentrate (PCC). This is a mixture of clotting factors, protein C and protein S. Trade names include Beriplex® or Octaplex®. They are very effective in immediately reversing warfarin but are very expensive. In most hospitals, they can only be administered after consultation with a haematologist.

Your hospital will have a set of guidelines and these should be followed carefully. If in doubt, get haematology advice.

Thromboprophylaxis

All patients should have a thrombosis assessment performed. Most hospitals have a checklist. Risk factors include significantly reduced mobility, a limb in plaster, has sustained trauma, is over 65, has comorbidities or a past history of thrombosis. These apply to almost all trauma patients!

Most hospitals use low molecular weight heparin (LMWH). Twelve hours must be left between the last dose and surgery, but check the departmental policy and if in doubt, ask.

Antibiotics

If the patient is admitted for treatment of infection, determine from your seniors whether or not they want antibiotics to be administered immediately. If they are planning to drain an abscess or washout a joint, they may request that antibiotics are held until intraoperative specimens have been obtained for culture. If the patient is septic or unwell, antibiotics should be given as soon as possible and blood cultures taken beforehand.

Consent

You should not take consent unless you have been specifically trained to do so and understand the procedure.

54 The operating theatre

Figure 54.1 Theatre layout

A typical orthopaedic theatre layout is shown. The patient enters from the clean corridor through the anaesthetic room. Surgery takes place in the central section of the operating theatre, beneath the laminar flow hood. Whilst surgery is in progress, staff should only enter the theatre through the anaesthetic or scrub room, and not through the main exit doors

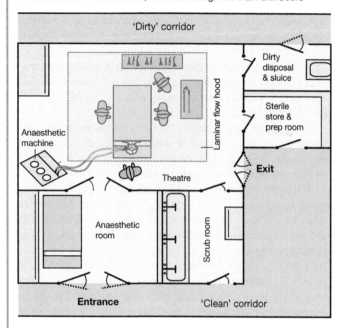

Figure 54.2 Laminar flow

In order to minimise airborne contaminants, the air is passed through very fine filters before being guided in a parallel stream by a perspex hood suspended from the ceiling. Staff should not enter the zone beneath the hood, marked by lines on the floor, unless they are scrubbed

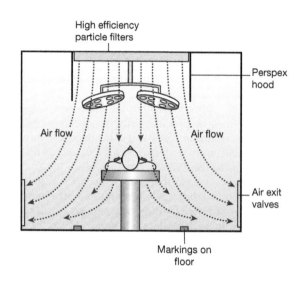

Figure 54.3 The WHO Surgical Safety Checklist is followed before and after every operation in order to minimise errors

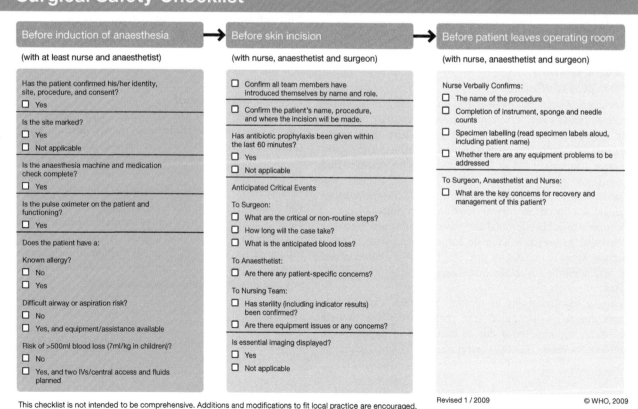

Theatre basics

Attending theatre is not optional! It is a vital part of your orthopaedic Foundation training. Even if you want to be a GP and have no desire ever to set foot in an operating theatre again, there is a shortlist of cases that you must see:
- **Total hip replacement**
- **Total knee replacement**
- **Fractured neck of femur operation (DHS or hemiarthroplasty)**
- **Long bone fracture fixation**

By getting involved, and making the right impression, you will be allowed to scrub in and learn suturing and other basic surgical skills.

In order to make the most of your time in theatre, take the following approach:
- Introduce yourself – there are two key players who will want to know who you are: the surgeon and the theatre sister. Find them at the beginning of the list.
- Know what's on the list – it does not look good if you turn up without knowing what cases are on the list! Lists are published the day before and are available from theatre reception.
- See patients preoperatively – the surgeon will see the patients before the list starts, to explain the operation and obtain consent. It is an important process and a valuable learning opportunity for you. Patients will normally come to a preoperative holding ward at 7.30 for a morning list, and at midday for an afternoon list.
- Read up on cases – if you are very keen and want to impress, read up on the cases beforehand. There are a variety of operative textbooks. *Campbells' Operative Orthopaedics* is the traditional tome, but illustrated lighter texts such as *Practical Procedures in Orthopaedic Trauma Surgery* by Giannoudis are also good.
- Ask questions: improve your new-found knowledge!

Sterility

In order to avoid the catastrophic consequences of infection in orthopaedics, there is a great emphasis on sterility. This is much more so than general surgery where the field is often contaminated by pus or faeces.

You must avoid contaminating the field, the instruments or yourself!

Blue or green

Never touch anything that is blue or green unless you are scrubbed. Be particularly careful with loose clothing brushing against the trolley.

Masks

Most contaminants in the air are borne upon exhaled breath. Once the sterile trays are opened, everyone in theatre should wear a mask.

Ventilation

Orthopaedic theatres have a laminar flow ventilation system. This comprises a set of very fine particle filters in the ceiling, through which clean air is pumped. A perspex frame suspended from the edges of the filter set guides the flow of air. Any disturbance of the air flow in this area risks contamination. Do not stand under the frame unless you are scrubbed. Do not open the outside doors into theatre once surgery has started. Enter instead through the anaesthetic room or the scrub room.

Scrub technique

If you have never scrubbed before, ask for assistance. If you think you have inadvertently contaminated yourself whilst donning gown or gloves, start again. Do not just ignore it! Generally speaking, most orthopaedic cases require you to wear two pairs of gloves. This offers protection from sharp instruments and spikes of bone, as well as allowing frequent changes of top gloves to prevent contamination.

Intraoperative etiquette

Ask if you can scrub in, as this affords you a better view and minimises the risk of contamination. Ask questions but be mindful of timing – if the surgeon is concentrating, it may be better to be quiet for a minute. Do not put your hands in the wound unless you have been given permission to do so.

Universal precautions

These are designed to avoid injury to yourself, your colleagues and the patient. Wearing eye protection and a mask is mandatory. All sharp instruments should be passed in a kidney dish. Do not re-sheath needles. When passing sutures back to the nurse, protect the tip with the needle-holder.

Needlestick injury

If you do sustain a needlestick injury, tell the theatre sister. Immediately descrub and wash your hand under running water, squeezing the wound to encourage bleeding. Fill in an incident form, contact occupational health and assess the risk of blood-borne disease.

The perioperative process

Time out

Before the start of surgery the whole surgical team stops and runs through a checklist. This is akin to the lists that pilots use when flying an aircraft. The patient's identity is checked, the operation site and consent are confirmed. Any special equipment or steps are identified. This is an important patient safety adjunct.

Anaesthetic

There are a variety of anaesthetic techniques, and it is important that you have a grasp of the underlying principles of each. Speak to the anaesthetist and try to spend some time in the anaesthetic room.

Tourniquet

An inflatable tourniquet is used to control bleeding in extremity surgery. The limb must first be exsanguinated. This is performed with an elasticated 'Esmarch' bandage or a pneumatic sausage-shaped 'Rhys-Davies' device. The cuff is then inflated to around 250 mmHg for the upper limb and 300 mmHg for the lower limb. If the cuff is too narrow, or the pressure insufficient to completely arrest arterial flow, the result is venous congestion and increased bleeding. Limb ischaemia results in accumulation of lactic acid and other products of metabolism. Tourniquets are applied for a maximum of 2 hours.

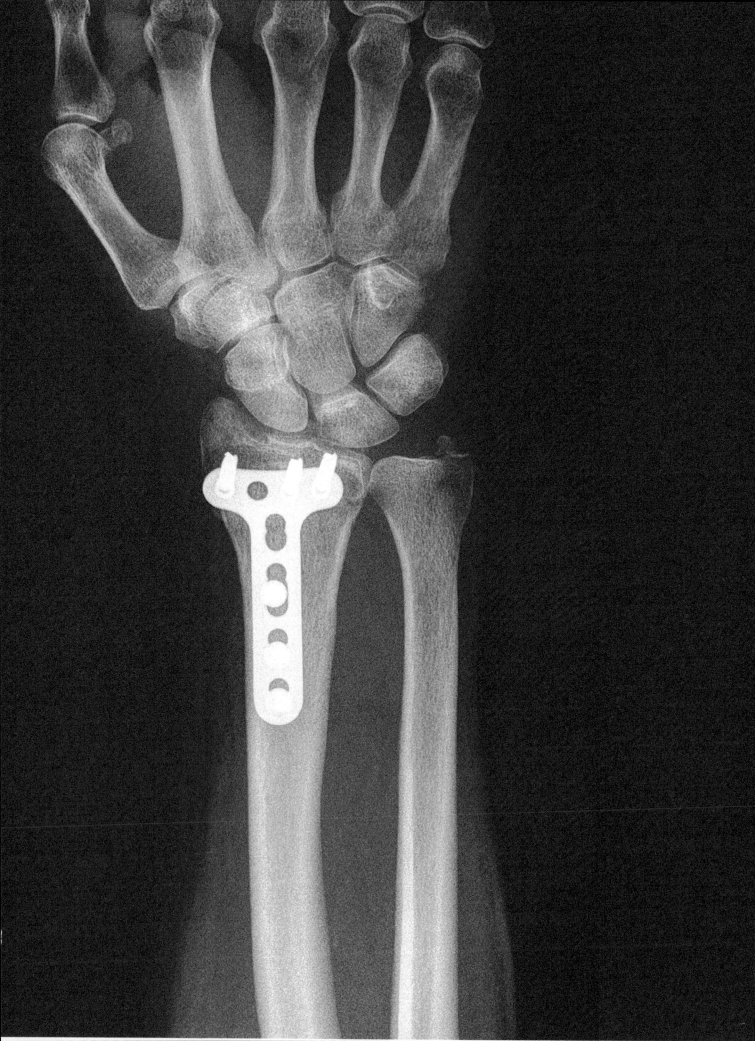

Practical procedures

Part 6

 Visit the companion website at www.ataglanceseries.com/TandO to test yourself on these topics.

55 Practical procedures 1

Figure 55.1 Haematoma block

For a distal radius fracture in an adult use 5 ml 0.5% bupivicaine and 5 ml lignocaine in a 10-ml syringe. A green needle inserted perpendicular to the skin will enter the fracture haematoma. The position is confirmed by aspirating blood mixed with fat globules, which rise to the top of the syringe

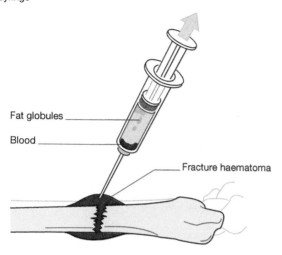

Fat globules

Blood

Fracture haematoma

Figure 55.2 Fracture reduction

Often periosteum is caught in the fracture site, which hampers reduction. Exaggerating the deformity whilst applying traction frees the periosteum and allow anatomical reduction

1 Periosteum caught in fracture

2 Exaggerating deformity frees periosteum

3 Anatomical reduction is then achieved

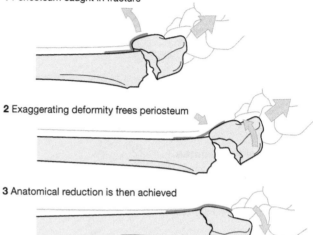

Figure 55.3 A below-elbow backslab requires 4–inch eight–ply plaster, cut as shown

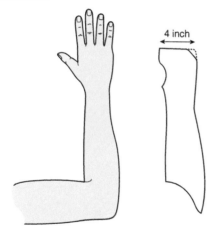

4 inch

Figure 55.4 Three point fixation

Moulding the plaster with pressure at three points, two dorsally and one volar, securely holds the fracture in position. Be careful only to use the flat of your hands as finger imprints can lead to pressure sores

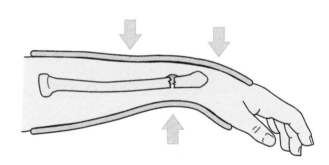

Figure 55.5 A below-knee backslab is composed of a 6-inch eight-ply slab and a 4-inch four-ply stirrup which adds stability

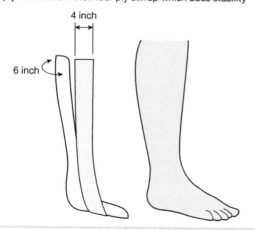

4 inch

6 inch

Figure 55.6 Manipulation of shoulder dislocation

Adequate analgesia is given. An assistant uses a folded sheet in the axilla as countertraction. Sustained in-line traction to the arm disimpacts the shoulder. Gentle internal and external rotation may be needed. As the shoulder reduces with a clunk, bring the arm across the body and secure with a splint

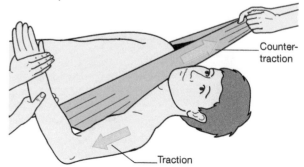

Counter-traction

Traction

Trauma and Orthopaedics at a Glance, First Edition. Henry Willmott.
© 2016 John Wiley & Sons, Ltd. Published 2016 by John Wiley & Sons, Ltd. Companion website: www.ataglanceseries.com/TandO

This chapter is not a substitute for proper teaching of these techniques. You must have adequate supervision by appropriately skilled individuals until you are competent.

Closed manipulation of a fracture

Consider the mechanism and reverse the causative force. Review the X-rays and visualise how you will manipulate the fracture fragments.

Ensure adequate analgesia (see below).

Apply longitudinal traction: this disimpacts fracture fragments, restores length and corrects angulation. Ask a colleague to apply counter-traction. Pull for several minutes to stretch tight periosteum and overcome the pull of muscles. Keep your arms outstretched and use your own bodyweight. Beware of shearing skin, especially in the elderly. Latex gloves may increase the risk of causing a skin tear.

Correct residual angulation with the heels of your hands, one below the fracture, the other distally. You may need to gently exaggerate the deformity to disimpact bone spikes or thick periosteum in children.

Apply a backslab, check neurovascular status and repeat X-rays.

Haematoma block

A useful way of providing analgesia without sedation is to inject local anaesthetic into the fracture haematoma. This is effective up to 8 hours after injury.

Sterility is essential. Clean the skin thoroughly.

Mix 10 mL of 50:50 0.5% bupivacaine and 2% lignocaine (lidocaine) for adults. The toxic dose of bupivacaine is 2 mg/kg, and that of lignocaine is 3 mg/kg.

Use a green needle to inject directly into the fracture haematoma. Aspirate. Dark blood mixed with fat globules that rise in the syringe indicate correct placement. The absence of fat may mean that you are in a vein – do not inject!

Inject 10 mL, apply a dressing and wait 10 minutes. Test gently before manipulation.

Plaster backslab application

Prepare: you need appropriate plaster, wool, bandage, tape and a bowl of lukewarm water. Hot water will make the plaster set too quickly and may burn the patient.

Protect the skin. Use a double layer of wool. Pay extra attention to bony prominences and pressure points. However, too much padding at the fracture site reduces the holding power of the cast.

Cut the plaster appropriately. Plaster slab comes in four layers. In adults a double- thickness (8 layers) is usually adequate. Use a 4-inch (10-cm) width for small wrists, 6-inch (15-cm) for larger wrists and 8-inch (20-cm) for lower limb casts.

Hold one end of the plaster tightly and dunk in the water, ensuring it is thoroughly saturated. Do not wring out too much water. It should be sloppy.

Apply to the limb and gently wrap with a bandage. Secure with tape. If you need to apply moulding force, use the heels of your hands, not fingertips, which can cause divots.

Ensure that the two sides of the back slab do not overlap each other. You need to maintain a section of soft bandage all the way along the cast to allow for swelling. Check neurovascular status and warn about signs of compartment syndrome.

Manipulation of shoulder dislocation

Carefully assess X-rays for the presence of a fracture.

Check and document the neurovascular status, including axillary nerve function.

Ensure adequate analgesia or sedation by an anaesthetist.

Get a colleague or nurse to provide counter-traction with a strip of collar and cuff or a bedsheet in the axilla.

Adduct the arm and apply longitudinal traction, maintaining a firm pull for 3–5 minutes (time yourself).

Gently internally and externally rotate the arm to disimpact a Hill–Sachs lesion. Do not force or twist!

The shoulder should reduce with a clunk. Bring the arm across the body to maintain the reduction. Apply a broad arm sling. Reassess neurovascular status and obtain X-rays including axillary view.

Failure is an indication for manipulation under general anaesthetic.

Practical procedures 2

Figure 56.1 Knee aspiration

The knee should be supported in 15–20° flexion with a pillow underneath. Set up a sterile field. Entry point is 1 cm above and 1 cm lateral to the patella. The needle is held at 45° in all places and advanced with continuous back-pressure on the plunger

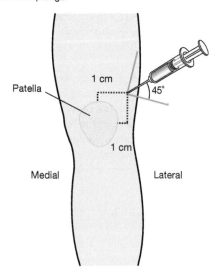

Figure 56.2 Types of suture

Braided and monofilament. Both are available in absorbable and non-absorbable materials

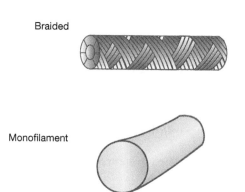

Figure 56.3 Suture techniques

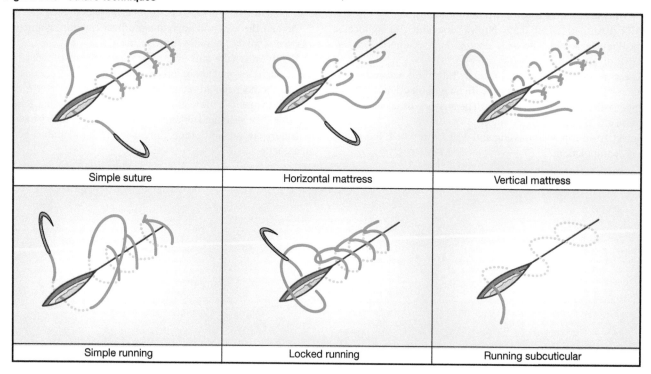

Trauma and Orthopaedics at a Glance, First Edition. Henry Willmott.
© 2016 John Wiley & Sons, Ltd. Published 2016 by John Wiley & Sons, Ltd. Companion website: www.ataglanceseries.com/TandO

Aspiration of a joint (knee)

Indications: diagnostic to exclude septic arthritis or crystal arthropathy; therapeutic for acute haemarthrosis or reactive effusion.

Contraindications: presence of a prosthetic joint (this should only be done in theatre), deranged clotting or high INR, overlying cellulitis.

You will need skin prep, a sterile wound pack, sterile gloves, a white needle, three or four 20-mL syringes, an adhesive dressing.

- Mark the skin: for the knee, palpate and draw the outline of the patella, the patellar tendon and the joint line.
- Choose your site: if the patient is comfortable with the knee in 15° flexion, support the knee with a pillow or blanket.
- Mark a horizontal line 1 cm above the superior pole of the patella and another perpendicular line 1 cm lateral to the patella. Where these two lines meet is the entry point.
- Use full aseptic precautions: wash your hands, use a sterile field, sterile gloves, proper skin prep such as chlorhexidine or Betadine®.
- Use a white or long green needle and insert it at 45° in all planes; aiming for the opposite wheel of the trolley is a helpful guide.
- Aspirate as you advance. You will feel a pop as you enter the joint and the syringe will fill with fluid. If you hit bone, it is either the patella or femur. Withdraw and redirect accordingly. The first syringe is your specimen.
- If there is a large effusion, keep the needle in situ and change to a new syringe. Keep aspirating until the knee is dry.
- Withdraw the needle and apply a dressing. A firm wool and crepe bandage may prevent a haemarthrosis from reaccumulating.

Typical aspirate appearance

Send the speciment for MC&S, including crystal microscopy. Inform the lab that it is on its way and ask them to call with the result.

Although not diagnostic, the typical appearance of different fluid specimens is given below:

- Gout is a yellow turbid fluid.
- A reactive effusion is a clear yellow.
- Infection is thick, turbid yellow or green fluid.
- Fracture results in a mixture of fat and blood.
- Plain blood may be due to deranged clotting.

Suturing

The best place to learn suturing is in theatre. You can practise on a banana skin or orange peel in your own time.

Suture materials

- Absorbable (Vicryl®) or non-absorbable (nylon).
- Monofilament (Monocryl®) or braided (Ethibond®).

Suture techniques

- Simple interrupted suture – commonly used for skin, removed after 10–14 days.
- Mattress suture (horizontal or vertical) – used in skin, to ensure eversion of the skin edge and to prevent tension.
- Simple running suture – commonly used in deep fascia.
- Locked running suture – sometimes used in skin or fascia to reduce the risk of the suture cutting out.
- Running subcuticular suture – commonly used with absorbable suture material to close skin, providing good cosmesis and avoiding the need to return for suture removal.

Index

Trauma and Orthopaedics at a Glance, First Edition. Henry Willmott.
© 2016 John Wiley & Sons, Ltd. Published 2016 by John Wiley & Sons, Ltd. Companion website: www.ataglanceseries.com/TandO